OVERCOMING
INSOMNIA

OVERCOMING INSOMNIA

A MEDICAL PROGRAM FOR PROBLEM SLEEPERS

by

Donald R. Sweeney, M.D., Ph.D.

G. P. PUTNAM'S SONS

The information contained in this book is the result of a careful review of the medical literature. However, new information is constantly becoming available and individual responses to specific treatments, methods, and medications vary widely from person to person. The reader is encouraged to consult with a physician in dealing with serious and persistent sleeping disorders and before taking any medication. The author and publisher specifically disclaim any adverse effect or unforeseen consequences resulting from the implementation of any information mentioned in this book.

G. P. Putnam's Sons
Publishers Since 1838
200 Madison Avenue
New York, NY 10016

Library of Congress Cataloging-in-Publication Data

Sweeney, Donald R., date.
    Overcoming insomnia: a medical program for problem sleepers / by
Donald R. Sweeney.—1st American ed.
        p.   cm.
    Bibliography: p.
    Includes index.
    ISBN 0-399-13405-0
        1. Insomnia—Treatment. I. Title.
    RC548.S93 1988
    616.8'49—dc19   88-18497 CIP

Book design by ARLENE GOLDBERG

Printed in the United States of America

1   2   3   4   5   6   7   8   9   10

*To the Clinical Staff at Fair Oaks Hospital,
which for the last decade has been a constant
source of support and encouragement.*

Contents

ACKNOWLEDGMENTS

I am especially grateful to Ron Schaumburg for his invaluable contribution to this book, which benefited enormously from his considerable talents.

In addition, I am indebted to my colleagues at Fair Oaks Hospital, including Mark S. Gold, M.D., A. Carter Pottash, M.D., and Andrew E. Slaby, M.D., Ph.D., M.P.H., for their professional and personal support.

My gratitude is also extended to the staff of The Putnam Publishing Group, and especially to my editor, Adrienne Ingrum, whose guidance and expert advice helped shape this book.

I am particularly indebted to my wife, Pamela, and my family for their love and support over the years.

Finally, I thank my patients, who have taught me a great deal about sleep disorders and the need for good, commonsense treatments.

Introduction

For most people, sleep brings rest and comfort, helping to reknit the fabric of their lives.

But for some—you, perhaps, or someone you love—sleep can be, literally, a nightmare. Tossing, turning, waking in the middle of the night can transform what should be a peaceful, restorative phase of the day into a debilitating, demoralizing, and potentially health-threatening debacle.

Over one third of the American population—roughly 80 million people—suffer at one time or another from some degree of sleep disturbance. And of that number, half consider their insomnia to be a serious problem. You may count yourself among them if you find that you

* lie in bed for what seems like hours, unable to drop off as your mind works over events of the day or anticipates tomorrow's crises
* sleep fitfully, your rest interrupted by snoring, twitching, or sudden awakenings
* have troubling dreams or "night panics"
* experience difficulty falling back asleep once awakened

* wake too early in the morning, staggering out of bed, never feeling really rested or caught up on your sleep
* struggle to stay awake during the day, yielding to the temptation to nap, or falling asleep uncontrollably

Perhaps your sleep disturbance is actually caused by another member of your household. Are you losing sleep over your husband's snoring? Do you wake up with bruised shins because your spouse kicks while asleep? Do your sleep patterns differ from those of your bedmate, turning the joy of sharing a bed into a headache?

Or perhaps you are the concerned parent of a child who wakes for any number of reasons during the night, or you are responsible for the care of an aging parent with sleep problems. There are sections of this book of special interest to you.

Without knowing it, you may be at risk from one of the more serious consequences of sleep disorders. Snoring, for example, may seem harmless, if annoying. But in severe cases it is a form of disrupted breathing that can cause high blood pressure, heart failure, even death. And the inability to sleep may be a symptom of other serious problems, including depression or other mental disorders. Such problems demand medical attention.

Experts estimate that sleepy employees cost businesses $70 billion a year in lost productivity, medical bills, and accidents—partially resulting from sleepy construction workers or forklift operators who crash their vehicles into walls, police officers falling asleep while waiting for traffic lights to change, or from salesmen who drop off to sleep in the middle of their pitch to a customer.

In 1987 authorities closed the Peach Bottom Power Station, a nuclear plant in Pennsylvania, because controllers were discovered sleeping during their night and weekend shifts. In another instance, an operator at a waste-treatment plant nodded off during his midnight shift and accidently dumped thousands of gallons of dangerous chemicals into a river. Sleepy pilots pose a special risk. The National Transportation Safety Board has determined that pilot fatigue was either the cause or at least a contributing factor in 69 plane accidents resulting in the deaths of 67 people between 1983 and 1986.

Clearly sleep disorders are a national concern.

Generally people refer to sleep disturbances under the collective term "insomnia." As you'll soon see, however, insomnia travels under many names and in many disguises. One purpose of this book is to help you recognize and identify the different types of insomnia and their causes—both physical and emotional—as a first step in achieving a good night's sleep. You'll discover a number of ways in which you can help yourself toward that goal, and you'll also learn when to turn to professionals for help.

That's the good news about insomnia—that help *is* available. Although sleep science is a relatively new medical discipline, considerable progress has been made over the past fifteen years in the way physicians diagnose and treat sleep disorders. Doctors are more aware of how their patients' lifestyles, emotions, even their jobs, interact to play significant roles in how well they rest at night. We know much more now about how such factors as exercise, diet, smoking, and intake of alcohol and caffeine affect people's ability to get a good night's sleep. And the exciting new science of chronobiology—how the various systems of the body act over the course of a day or a year—has much to teach us about sleep.

Over the years, as a psychiatrist, I've met and treated thousands of patients of virtually every age and walk of life. I've found that, to one extent or another, disturbed sleep may be a part of just about every medical or psychiatric condition. One fact I've observed in practice is that "insomnia," in and of itself, is seldom the problem. Rather, it is a symptom of a deeper disruption in the patient's mental or physical well-being.

My approach as a physician is to begin with a careful assessment of patients and their overall patterns, not just of sleeping but of waking, working, and interacting with others. In order to do so I obtain a detailed personal and family history, review the results of a thorough physical examination, and order the diagnostic and laboratory tests that I feel are crucial to understanding the underlying nature of the problem. I have learned the value of asking probing questions and drawing the patient out on topics that, while possibly uncomfortable, may provide invaluable insight into his or her situation. It has often turned out that the solution to a difficulty lies in clues provided by seemingly irrelevant bits of data about someone's style of living or working.

Only after I've gathered as much information as possible do I begin to outline a therapeutic approach. Sometimes I've found that the mere act of explaining some of the basic facts about the physical realities of sleep, its patterns and processes, can do a great deal to set the patient on the road to recovery. That, in fact, is part of my intention in writing this book.

Depending on the nature of the sleep disorder, treatments, many of them only recently developed, are now available which range from simple relaxation techniques to "time-shifting," and from psychological counseling to surgery. And it may be reassuring to know that sometimes the simplest, least expensive treatments are the most effective.

Amazingly, I've found that in some cases, opening or closing a window may make all the difference. In others, going to bed an hour later may actually make one sleep better and feel more refreshed. And you may be surprised to learn that "sleeping pills"—over-the-counter formulations as well as prescription drugs—may often be the wrong solution and may actually *contribute* to a sleeping problem.

It may be true, as some doctors are fond of saying, that "no one ever died from lack of sleep." Nor, for that matter, has insomnia ever been shown to cause heart attacks, strokes, or cancer, or even simpler afflictions like lines on the face or dark rings under the eyes. But it is also true that lack of sleep can weaken the body's systems, including the immune system, and put strain on the organs, making one more susceptible to attacks of infection, disease, and other infirmities, including depression.

Therefore your sleep problems *can and must be dealt with* if you are to live a happy and fulfilled existence. The fact that you are reading this book is a positive sign that you take your problem seriously enough to seek answers. While it is possible your insomnia is only temporary—the result of a change in lifestyle or a recent emotional disturbance—it is also possible there is a hidden medical cause which a professional will be able to recognize and help you resolve.

My primary goal in this book is to aid you in assessing your own situation in order to recognize the type of sleep disturbance that affects you or your loved one, and to guide you toward the treatment approach most likely to put your mind—and your body—at rest.

As we proceed you'll get a glimpse into the night world contained within our brains and our bodies, and you'll learn some fascinating things about sleep and sleepers.

For what may be the first time, you are holding in your hands a book whose main purpose is to put you to sleep.

1

Assessing Your Sleep Pattern

Like most physicians I've grown accustomed to having people accosting me in search of free medical advice—especially when they suffer, or think they suffer, from insomnia. Invariably these people are disappointed when I suggest they come to see me, or another physician, in a professional setting. But as you can see from the length of this book, the subject of insomnia is a very complex one: I would not be helping people by giving quick suggestions. In fact, I would need to ask many questions before I could properly address their concerns.

In the following section, I have included the types of questions I might ask in order to diagnose your sleep disorder correctly. And if I determined that you were suffering from a true sleep disorder, I would use your answers to these questions in formulating the most effective treatment plan for you.

Your accurate responses to such questions can make a world of difference in identifying the nature of your insomnia. Perhaps you drag yourself out of bed in the morning and complain that you "didn't sleep a wink all night." But do you actually lie in bed, eyes open, staring at the ceiling, bedeviled by tangled, troubling thoughts? Or do you sleep intermittently, fitfully, or in brief, unrestful snatches?

Do you have trouble falling asleep initially, or do you awaken in the middle of the night, unable to return to sleep?

Is there some emotional disturbance—suppressed anger, for example, or recent grief—that may be contributing to your problem?

The first step in understanding the nature of your sleeping problem and its possible causes and developing a strategy that will provide the quickest, most effective results is to assess the nature of your sleep patterns. You'll need to evaluate your current personal habits, such as diet, exercise, and lifestyle, and you'll want to note your past sleep patterns. Keeping a sleep diary (which might more accurately be called a "noctuary") will also help to define your patterns.

At the very least, just thinking about the questions will strengthen your awareness of your sleep problem, and the deeper awareness you garner from your answers will prove especially helpful in establishing your own treatment program.

The first assessment, Current Health and Lifestyle, is designed to uncover the recent factors that may be causing your insomnia. How many cigarettes you smoke or whether or not you take over-the-counter medications, for example, may seem irrelevant to your sleep problems. In reality, however, many of our daily habits and practices, while seemingly harmless, can cause insomnia. The use of cigarettes or certain medications can actually result in disturbed sleep. So answer all the questions carefully, no matter how unusual.

The second part, Your Sleep History, focuses directly on your personal sleep patterns. The purpose of these questions is to find out if your insomnia is recent or long-term, and if there might be a physical or psychological reason for the condition.

Your third "assignment," the Sleep Diary, will provide a record of the actual number of hours you sleep each night, as well as a log of the factors that may influence your sleep, such as alcohol, coffee, and cigarette consumption. Often people are surprised to find out how many cups of coffee they drink—and when they drink them.

Remember to answer each of the following questions carefully. Jot down your answers in a notebook—you'll find it extremely helpful to refer to your responses as you read this book. The questions may seem like a lot of work, but overcoming insomnia is not an easy task. Your direct, active involvement in obtaining a correct diagnosis and implementing proper treatment for your sleep disorder is essential.

CURRENT HEALTH AND LIFESTYLE

Rate your overall health on a scale of 1 (poor) to 10 (excellent).

List any chronic diseases or conditions (asthma, allergies, arthritis, ulcer, back pain, high blood pressure, diabetes, etc.).

List past major illnesses, injuries, and hospitalizations, including approximate dates the problem began, treatment, date of recovery, any lingering symptoms.

List any medical problems within the last year or so, including any seasonal problems such as allergies, mood swings, etc.

Are you seeing a psychiatrist or any other type of counselor? If yes, for how long? Describe any therapeutic program you are following (drugs, counseling, etc.).

If you think you are overweight, indicate by how many pounds.

Indicate any findings from a recent physical examination, such as blood pressure, heart rate, and overall health.

Rate your overall energy level on a scale of 1 (constantly fatigued) to 10 (constantly energetic).

If you currently work, how many hours a day? Do you consider yourself a workaholic?

Do you smoke? If so, how many packs a day?

Do you drink? If so, how many drinks per week?

Do you regularly drink a nightcap to help you sleep? If so, how many drinks?

How much of the following do you consume on the average each day:

coffee (caffeinated)   (6-ounce cups)
coffee (decaffeinated)   (6-ounce cups)

tea (caffeinated)	(6-ounce cups)
tea (herbal or decaffeinated)	(6-ounce cups)
caffeinated soft drinks	(6-ounce cups)
chocolate	(2-ounce bars)

Rate your general eating habits on a scale of 1 (irregular eating schedule; poor nutritional balance) to 10 (regular schedule, balanced diet).

Within the last thirty days, have you taken:

Any prescription drugs for sleep? List the drug, dosage, and regimen.

Any non-prescription sleeping aids? List name, dosage, active ingredient if known.

Any other medication for any medical problem? List all drugs, injections, dosages, and regimens, and whether drug is prescription or over-the-counter.

Any illegal drugs (marijuana, cocaine, hallucinogenics, amphetamines)?

Do you exercise regularly? If so, indicate the types of exercise, frequency, your typical regimen, time of day of exercise.

Do you practice any form of structured relaxation exercises (including transcendental meditation, yoga, Zen, etc.)? If so, describe your regimen.

How many people share your living quarters? What ages?

Do you have a bedmate (spouse, lover)?

How many times per month do you have sexual intercourse?

Rate your sexual activity on a scale of 1 (very unsatisfactory) to 10 (very satisfactory).

Describe any sexual problems such as impotence, frigidity, etc.

Do you experience headaches on waking? How often?

Do you feel you are not able to think as quickly or as effectively as you used to?

Do others describe you as growing increasingly irritable or short-tempered?

Rate yourself from 1 to 10 on the following traits:

1	10
Worried	Carefree
Angry	Good-natured
Competitive	Laid-back
Aggressive	Relaxed
Impatient	Patient
Compulsive	Spontaneous
Depressed	Happy
Excitable	Calm
Argumentative	Agreeable
Easily upset	Patient
Suspicious	Trusting

How do you express your anger? Sadness? Love?

How do you respond to pressure?

As a rule, do you find it easy to confide in other people?

Do you take vacations regularly?

SLEEP HISTORY

What is your general attitude about sleep? (That is, do you look forward to going to sleep or do you dread the experience?)

Describe your sleep. Is it peaceful? Traumatic? Filled with unpleasant memories or associations?

Describe any sleep problems you remember from your childhood.

Describe any sleep problems experienced by members of your family (insomnia, sleepwalking, excessive daytime sleepiness, etc.).

Rate the degree of overall satisfaction you feel with your sleep pattern on a scale from 1 (very dissatisfied) to 10 (very satisfied).

How many times a week do you experience difficulty sleeping?

Is your sleep difficulty improving, worsening, or remaining fairly constant?

When did you first experience difficulty sleeping (within the last month, within the last six months, within the last year, or over a year ago)?

Do you ascribe any particular cause to your sleeping difficulty (i.e., emotional strain, physical trauma)?

What time do you usually try to go to bed?

Is your bedtime regular or does it vary by an hour or more each night?

Which of the following more closely describes your situation: I usually go to bed when I feel sleepy, regardless of what time it is. I go to bed at the same time whether I'm sleepy or not.

How long do you usually lie in bed before you fall asleep (less than ten minutes, less than thirty minutes, over thirty minutes)?

What time do you usually try to awaken?

Does your sleep pattern differ on weekends? How (time of rising and going to bed, hours of sleep, etc.)?

Do you notice a difference in your sleep satisfaction on weekends compared with weekdays?

Rate your usual state of mind when you go to bed on a scale from 1 (anxious) to 10 (relaxed).

Rate your usual state of mind during the day on the same scale.

Rate the way you feel upon rising on a scale from 1 (very sleepy) to 10 (extremely refreshed).

After waking in the morning, how many minutes does it take you to begin functioning normally (less than ten minutes, less than thirty minutes, more than thirty minutes)?

Do you feel confused or "drunk" on waking? How often?

How much sleep do you usually get each night?

Counting any naps, how many hours a day do you sleep?

Do you have a bedtime ritual? If so, describe it (having a snack, checking the house, brushing teeth, bathing, watching a certain TV program, arranging bedclothes, laying out clothes for the next day, etc.).

Do you feel that any aspect of your work intrudes on your sleep? (For example, do you bring work home at night? Do you work in your bedroom just before sleeping? Do you ruminate about problems to be solved the following day?)

Do you awaken during the night? How many times? How much time in total are you awake?

If you awaken, are you usually able to return to sleep within five minutes?

If you are unable to return to sleep, what do you do (lie in bed, get up, read, eat, etc.)?

Do you awaken too early in the morning? If so, what do you do (get up, lie in bed, etc.)?

Do you feel excessively sleepy during the day? At any particular or predictable time?

Do you nap during the day? How many times? How long? Do you feel refreshed after napping?

Do you experience difficulty breathing during the day?

Do you ever awaken from shortness of breath? How often?

Do you snore? Does your bed partner complain about your snoring?

Do you know if your legs kick or twitch during the night?

Do you perspire excessively at night?

Answer the following questions on a scale from 1 (never) to 10 (every day).

Do you fall asleep:

When inactive
While watching television

While reading
While talking to other people
On the job
During entertainment events (movies, sports, etc.)
When you particularly want to stay awake
When emotionally aroused or excited

Under normal driving conditions, have you ever had to stop driving because of excessive sleepiness? Did you stop driving for several hours or only for a short time?

Do you ever fall down or feel weak when you are angry or when you laugh? (Falling down or muscle weakness following an emotional outburst may be a feature of narcolepsy. See Chapter 6.)

SLEEP DIARY

Maintain this diary regularly for the next three weeks. If you can do so without causing any disruption in your sleep routine, answer the following questions before going to sleep; if it suits your schedule better, answer them as soon as possible the next morning. Remember, record your answers in a notebook along with the responses to the first two questionnaires.

Coffee consumption (before 6 P.M.):

Coffee consumption (after 6 P.M.):

Cigarettes (before 6 P.M.):

Cigarettes (after 6 P.M.):

Alcohol consumption (before 6 P.M.):

Alcohol consumption (after 6 P.M.):

Prescription and over-the-counter medication (before 6 P.M.):

Prescription and over-the-counter medication (after 6 P.M.):

General ability to function, A.M. (scale 1–10):

General concentration, A.M. (scale 1–10):

General ability to function, P.M. (scale 1–10):

General concentration, P.M. (scale 1–10):

Describe any daytime sleepiness (intensity, time of day, etc.):

Stressful events: Describe:

Emotional events: Describe:

General mood during the day:

Naps: Number, time of day, total time today:

Total twenty-four-hour sleep time including naps:

Exercise: Regimen, time of day:

Dinnertime:

Snacks since dinner (including when eaten):

Activities from dinner to bedtime:

Presleep ritual: Describe:

Any sleeping pills? Describe:

Time you got into bed:

Bedtime mood (anxious, happy, etc.):

Sleepiness (scale 1–10):

Answer these questions on rising:

Time of waking:

Time of rising:

Approximate time you fell asleep:

Total hours in bed:

Total hours asleep:

Awaken before or with alarm?

Wakenings: Number:

Total time awake:

What did you do if awake?

Quality of sleep (scale 1–10)

Energy level on rising (scale 1–10)

The Next Step

You may not realize it now, but by answering the above questions and by beginning your sleep diary, you have taken an extremely important—perhaps the most important—step toward achieving a good night's sleep. You have begun the process of identifying the nature of your sleep disorder and the health, lifestyle, and personal history factors that may be causing it. Armed with the information you provide, you or your doctor will be well on the way to overcoming your insomnia.

For example, in the Current Health and Lifestyle assessment you may have answered that you regularly exercise prior to going to bed, while in the Sleep History you may have noted that you always go to bed at the same time and that you frequently find yourself lying in bed for over an hour before falling asleep. From these responses I might conclude that it is your habit of exercising prior to bedtime that is interfering with your sleep. Many people believe that exercising before bed makes sleeping easier, but as you will see in Chapter 8, this is not true. Other areas of the assessment, such as cigarette smoking and alcohol consumption, will also be covered in subsequent chapters.

In the next chapter we'll follow your personal sleep assessment with a discussion of the different types of sleep disorders as well as the physical and psychological conditions that may be at the root of your problem.

2

Why You Aren't Getting a Good Night's Sleep

Like many of you I love a good mystery novel. Piecing together the clues, trying to discern the real culprit from the pretenders, has kept me awake on many nights as I struggled with the temptation to turn to the last page. In a way being a doctor is very much like reading a mystery: We never have as much information as we would like, and sometimes, just when we are absolutely positive that we know who (or what) did it, we get our biggest surprise. Some of you may have dreamed of being a doctor; I, on the other hand, have always wanted to be the next Dick Francis or Robert Ludlum. For now, however, I must be content with being a doctor. Unfortunately, doctors cannot turn to the last page to find the solution to the whodunit.

Instead, we must rely a great deal upon the information you—the patient or members of the patient's family—provide. This is especially important since in sleep disorders, unlike most other areas of medicine, there are no readily available diagnostic tests like the X ray to guide us. Thus the information furnished by the previous chapter's self-assessment is crucial to a doctor's diagnosis.

It is also important that we be precise in the definitions of sleep disorders. Only with this precision can we begin to eliminate some of the confusion that surrounds the subject and design a therapeutic approach that has a hope of succeeding.

Clearly, confusion does exist. In a poll conducted by Stanford University, 4.3 percent of respondents described themselves as "insomniacs." At first glance, this low number would seem to belie the statement I made in my introduction, that as many as one out of three people in this country experience difficulty sleeping. But numbers and surveys can be deceiving. In this case the same Stanford survey went on to report that 38 percent of the group also declared that they had problems with at least one of the following: falling asleep, getting back to sleep after awakening during the night, awakening too early, and daytime tiredness. Strange, isn't it? Few claimed to be "insomniacs," but many suffered from the very symptoms that define insomnia.

With that in mind, then, let me try to clarify the terms I'll be using throughout this book in order to establish what a sleep disorder is and is not. These definitions are based on a consensus of doctors and psychiatrists and are widely used in diagnosis and treatment.

The Definitions of Sleep Disorders

"Insomnia," as reflected by the results of the Stanford poll, is a term broadly used to mean any form of sleep disorder. Specifically, however, it refers simply to the inability to sleep; its Latin roots mean "without sleep." Thus insomnia is just one form of sleep disorder. Sleep disorders can range from difficulty falling asleep to difficulty staying awake during the day. Those who analyze and treat sleep disorders break the subject down into subcategories, each with its own distinctive pattern of causes, symptoms, and consequences. Briefly, these categories of sleep disorders are:

* **Disorders of initiating and maintaining sleep (sometimes abbreviated DIMS):** DIMS is actually the technical term for what most people mean when they speak of insomnia. This term includes problems with falling asleep and problems staying asleep once sleep has been achieved. For example, you might lie in bed for an hour or more, unable to drop off, or you might snore so loudly as to awaken yourself.

* **Disorders of excessive somnolence (DOES; also called hypersomnia):** These disorders cause people to feel sleepy during the day or to feel unrested and less able to function. Included in this group are such illnesses as narcolepsy and sleep apnea, which result in insufficient sleep.
* **Disorders of the sleep-wake schedule (DSWS):** These problems stem from a variety of obvious causes, including jet lag and odd work shifts, or they may be the result of serious internal disruptions in an individual's biological clock (also called "circadian rhythms").
* **Parasomnias:** These are problems not with sleep itself but associated with, and disruptive of, sleep. Examples include sleepwalking, bed-wetting, and nightmares.

How frequently does each of these types of sleep disorder occur? According to the American Psychiatric Association, hypersomnia, or daytime sleepiness, is actually, and perhaps surprisingly, more prevalent than insomnia, the nighttime inability to sleep. Disorders of excessive sleepiness are found in roughly 50 percent of patients seeking help. Disorders of initiating and maintaining sleep account for approximately 30 percent, while parasomnias occur in 18 percent. Disorders of the sleep-wake schedule are a distinct minority at 2 percent, but that figure may change as scientists learn more about the hidden world of circadian rhythms.

From the above, then, "difficulty sleeping" obviously does not mean the occasional troubled night resulting from temporary discomfort, such as unfamiliar surroundings or uncooperative sheets and pillows. Nor does it refer to nights affected by short-term anxiety, caused perhaps by apprehension about the next day's final exam or annual salary review. I exclude too a night when a relatively minor physical ailment—an ankle sprained during a game of touch football or a nagging cough—keeps us awake. All of us go through nights when, for one obvious and short-lived reason or another, sleep simply will not descend on us. If we were to include such unpleasant but transient moments in our definition of sleep disorders, then the incidence among the population would undoubtedly equal 100 percent.

By now it should be clear that insomnia itself is not so much a specific disorder as it is a symptom which arises from one or more underlying psychiatric or medical pathologies and which should alert victims to a disruption in their normal physiological functioning. Similarly, insomnia may be the result of a disruption in lifestyle or living environment. As many as 60 to 80 percent of cases are psychological in origin, arising after stressful or traumatic events such as divorce, the death of a loved one, the loss of a job, or a move to a new city. Thus you may complain to your doctor of "insomnia," but after thorough examination the doctor may decide to treat you for anything from ulcers to depression. Only after the cause of troubled sleep has been addressed will the symptoms begin to dissipate.

With our definitions in mind, then, let me restate the point made earlier, that each year about a third of the people in the United States experience a period of prolonged sleep disturbance serious enough to disrupt their mental or physical well-being and affect their performance, to one degree or another, during their waking hours. Many of these disturbances are the result of physical or emotional illnesses and would likely respond to medical treatment. However, only about half of those suffering from a sleep disturbance as defined above consider their problem to be serious. And those who actually seek the advice of a physician represent an even smaller—but still significant—number; some estimates put the figure at 10 million out of the estimated 30 to 40 million cases per year.

Who Suffers from Sleep Disorders?

The likelihood of suffering from a sleep disturbance increases with age. In one survey almost 40 percent of persons over the age of fifty reported insomnia to be a current problem. And, according to one leading sleep researcher, 99 percent of the elderly experience disrupted sleep. (Generally, younger patients—those under the age of forty—suffer from difficulty in falling asleep; problems such as nighttime wakening or early-morning insomnia tend to occur in older patients.) Typically, insomnia is more prevalent among women and also among people who lack certain psychosocial advantages, such as adequate income, housing, or prestige, which in more fortunate individuals can help shore up any flagging sense of self-esteem. Single people reported more sleep problems than married ones, according to a Gallup poll (despite the fact that couples must contend with such hassles as snoring, twitching, and battling over blankets). As with some other medical conditions, women are twice as likely as men to seek help for their insomnia; similarly, they are twice as likely to have sleeping pills prescribed for them.

Some physicians—including me—fear that the accelerating pace of modern life may lead to a worsening of the problem. Today the drive to succeed at our careers, with our families, and in our social lives is higher, perhaps, than at any other time in history. As we come to demand more of ourselves and of others, society as a whole will become less tolerant of "sleepy" people, those who appear lazy by taking things at a more relaxed pace or who seem too willing to settle for less. This intolerance will turn up the pressure on these hapless souls, increasing their level of stress and leading to a higher rate of stress-related conditions such as insomnia, ulcers, high blood pressure, and heart disease.

It is impossible to overemphasize the need to *prevent* sleep disorders from developing. Should our efforts at prevention fail, however, it is important to recognize and treat the causes as promptly as possible. Left to fester, a sleep disturbance can grow from a transient annoyance to a major source of distress in and of itself. In those cases the patient may come to perceive the insomnia as a distinct disorder, which, as I've explained, it is not. Poor sleep thus becomes, in a very real sense, a bad habit, a form of self-destructive learned behavior whose ultimate consequences may include increased anxiety and depression. Should that occur, the insomnia may persist long after the precipitating cause has been eliminated.

For those people who believe that there is a chemical solution to every problem, I'm afraid I bear bad news: No pill yet invented will cure a case of chronic insomnia. Despite this Americans continue to spend millions of dollars on sleep remedies, both prescription and over-the-counter, in their quest for a good night's sleep. Over 20 million prescriptions for "sleeping pills" are written in the United States each year; an even larger number of over-the-counter sleep aids is sold. More drugs are used in connection with sleep than for any other therapeutic purpose. As we'll see, use of these drugs often fails to address the cause of the insomnia and can worsen the problem while preventing more effective therapies from being tried.

One point should be stressed about the treatment of sleep disorders. Insomnia, hypersomnia, and the other manifestations of disturbed sleep are not the exclusive province of any one medical discipline. Sleep disturbance may result from a neurological disorder or from some organic flaw in the cardiovascular or intestinal system. Conversely, the core of insomnia may lie buried within a traumatic emotional experience suffered by the victim years before its symptoms become manifest. The patient may confess to feelings of anxiety or excessive worry, but analysis conducted in a sleep laboratory may reveal the presence of severely disordered nocturnal breathing. Thus treatment of serious sleep disruption may require the services of many branches of medicine—internal, neurologic, and psychiatric; forms of therapy may range from psychological counseling to behavior modification, from drugs to surgery. For particularly recalcitrant cases, several approaches may need to be tried sequentially or simultaneously. I say this not to frighten but to reassure: for those who seek it, help—effective, methodical, multifaceted help—is available.

Let's look more closely now at the different common causes of insomnia—psychological, medical, and lifestyle.

PSYCHOLOGICAL CAUSES OF INSOMNIA

By far the most frequent source of insomnia is some form of mental or emotional disquiet. Since one primary biological reason for sleep is to provide the brain with a chance to rest, it is perhaps not surprising that one consequence of a troubled mind should be troubled sleep.

I must hasten to point out that in using such terms as "mental disquiet" or "psychological disturbance" I am not suggesting, by any stretch of the imagination, that people with insomnia are thereby crazy, or that their sleep troubles are "all in their minds." Quite the contrary. Insomnia is a very real, and very widely experienced, phenomenon. Insomniacs really do sleep less than other people, as measured not just by their own perceptions but clinically and scientifically in sleep laboratories. Nor do victims of insomnia have unrealistic expectations or beliefs about what constitutes a good night's sleep; studies have shown that insomniacs desire only the same amount of sleep as other people.

While it is true that insomnia is a feature of a number of severe mental disorders, including clinical depression, it may also appear when a psychologically healthy person's life is unusually stressful or tension-filled. Often people with sleep disorders have endured troubling situations over which they had no control—an unhappy home life during childhood, for example. And the increasing pressure and pace of today's society adds to everyone's mental load. The primary purpose of labeling insomnia as largely psychiatric in origin is not to suggest that the disorder is illusory or that its victims are mentally disturbed but to call attention to the types of therapy that have the greatest chance of succeeding.

With that in mind, then, let me proceed to describe some of the behavioral patterns and mental attitudes that are frequently associated with insomnia. Perhaps you will recognize one or more of these traits in yourself or in a loved one who suffers from sleepless nights. If so, you will be better able to focus on the cause of the problem—the first step toward resolving it.

Generally, studies indicate that patients with chronic insomnia report fewer positive experiences during childhood. This can mean a number of things. Perhaps their parents quarreled constantly or criticized harshly. Possibly there was violence or abuse in the home. There may have been few rewarding family relationships: no siblings, or too many; lack of an extended family; little or no time to interact with parents due to conflicting or demanding work schedules. Perhaps the family moved often, making it difficult to find and sustain friendships or to establish one's role in a school or a community. In such cases, people often fail to develop a healthy sense of self-esteem. As a consequence, they find it difficult as time goes on to sustain healthy interpersonal relationships. They may also fail to develop adequate methods of coping with stress: in some cases, they may avoid confrontation rather than meet a problem or an opponent head-on.

One commonly found trait among insomniacs is their tendency to internalize their emotions. Perhaps as children they were discouraged from expressing their feelings or were ridiculed for their attitudes and behavior. In time, then, these people may have learned to suppress their feelings of anger or hostility or sadness—or even joy—either through habit or as a mechanism of defense against hurt or shame. Common wisdom and scientific research support the view that failure to express such feelings can result in physical as well as emotional consequences. Insomnia, as we are seeing, is one of them.

Emotional suppression is a vicious circle. To illustrate, let me relate an anecdote about a patient I'll call Howard. This thirty-eight-year-old man worked at two jobs in an effort to support his four children. Howard suffered from chronic gastrointestinal disorders—perhaps one reaction to the stress he felt. In one capacity, as an assembly-line worker at a leather-goods plant, he was called upon to stand for long, uninterrupted hours operating a drill punch. One day, plagued by diarrhea, he needed to leave his post virtually every hour. His boss, who had always been difficult to deal with, grew increasingly frustrated with each absence, since it disrupted the flow of work for the entire assembly line. Throughout the day, in the presence of other employees, the boss hurled insults and snide remarks at Howard, ridiculing his condition and mocking his perceived weakness. Howard confided to me later that he grew increasingly angry and had thoughts of violence toward the man, but he suppressed them since he depended so heavily on his job. Within a week Howard's condition grew worse, and he was fired for "laziness." The loss of income preyed on his mind, and Howard began to suffer a string of sleepless nights.

You can see the pattern: Financial pressure caused Howard to work doubly hard. The added strain of a difficult boss exacerbated his gastrointestinal disorder, which, ironically, made the boss even harder to deal with. The escalating conflict led to Howard's termination, which in turn led to increasing financial pressure and, ultimately, to insomnia.

Obviously a complex case such as Howard's could not be resolved overnight. Merely advising Howard that he should have told his boss off or channeled his hostility into some constructive activity would have served no purpose. In the course of our

conversations, however, this patient began to realize that he had
been carrying a huge emotional burden by himself. Somewhere
along the line he had been taught that to complain or ask for
support from another person, especially his wife, was a sign of
weakness which would mark him as unfit to support a family.

I explained to Howard that suppressing emotions has the unpleasant, and potentially dangerous, consequence of stimulating
that part of our nervous system, the autonomic system, which is
responsible for our unconscious activities such as heartbeat and
breathing. We might feel anger and want to lash out at someone.
If we trap that energy within, however, our bodies must find a
way to expend it; they do so by increasing the activity in the
systems not in our conscious control, including those regulating
muscle tension and the constriction of blood vessels. Such activity tends to reach its peak at the end of the day, with the result
that it disrupts our ability to sleep.

With encouragement, Howard began to communicate more
openly with his family. As a result several things happened:
ways were found to cut back on expenses and reduce the financial pressure to some extent. His wife took a part-time job, something she had wanted to do anyway but had not acted on for fear
it would threaten Howard's position as breadwinner. Recently
Howard reported that while things are by no means easy, by
letting his family know the realities of his situation he discovered a previously unknown dimension of their love and support.
His insomnia, I should add, has abated considerably.

Howard's story illustrates another factor of sleep disturbance:
Its appearance is often connected to the occurrence of stressful
life events. Such events can produce anxiety or depression and
can cause us to ruminate about the situation in a cyclic and
increasingly frustrating pattern. When people begin to have disturbed sleep, they also begin to worry that they won't get enough
rest. In other words, ironically, they lose sleep worrying about
whether they are going to lose sleep. Unless they realize that this
pattern exists, either through their own efforts or with professional help, such people will continue to suffer.

As a rule, victims of insomnia reveal similar patterns of behavior. At bedtime, for example, the tensions of the day have accumulated to a fever pitch. Thoughts of work, health, personal
problems, even death, predominate. They awaken feeling even

worse: sleepy, groggy, tired physically as well as mentally. They slog through the day worried, tense, anxious, and irritable. They may describe themselves as nervous, lonely, or lacking in self-confidence. In extreme cases they may be depressed and report that they fear they will lose control of themselves. Many feel that their situation is "hopeless."

I'd like to expand briefly on the association between insomnia and thoughts of death. Some experts feel that fear of death may underlie all forms of insomnia. I remember the little bedtime prayer I used to say as a child: "Now I lay me down to sleep, I pray the Lord my soul to keep. If I die before I wake, I pray the Lord my soul to take." How strange that so strong a connection between death and sleep should be forged in the prayers of children. For some the negative associations of sleep are extended to everything connected with the bedroom: darkness, pillows, even a toothbrush. One insomniac patient of mine noticed that his heart began to race as soon as he started to put on his pajamas. A small but significant element of his therapy was to encourage him to sleep in the nude.

An interesting complication I've observed in some cases of insomnia is the patient's interaction with other members of the family. For example, a patient I'll call Joanne seemed reluctant to adopt any of the treatments I suggested for her problem. On digging further I realized that through her suffering from sleeplessness, Joanne was able to extract a high degree of sympathy and support from her family. She had somehow learned, subliminally, that by means of her illness she could manipulate others into expressing love and concern, thus reinforcing her own sense of self-worth. The reason for her reluctance to be cured became obvious: Without the illness that made people feel sorry for her she would lose a source of emotional support on which she had come to depend.

Conversely, there are family members who unintentionally reinforce the patient's insomnia by the attention they pay to it. Their own need to feel important or helpful to the victim is served when they express concern or sympathy. Unconsciously they create a situation whereby they encourage the patient to suffer from insomnia in order to satisfy their own need to be needed.

One other trait common to insomnia victims is their tendency to exaggerate their symptoms. I hasten to repeat that the problem is very real, but their perception of its severity may be somewhat skewed. For example, I have often heard patients say they get only four or five hours of sleep, only to find that when assessed in a sleep clinic they sleep for six or seven hours. Similarly, a patient with delayed onset of sleep may say she lies awake for an hour before dropping off, when a study finds the period of time to be fifteen minutes or less. In my practice, then, I make it a point to get as accurate a description of the patient's sleeping problem as possible, by using the types of questions found in the self-assessment section, pages 16 through 23. This may mean enlisting the aid of the bed partner or, in extreme cases, referring the patient for overnight analysis in a sleep laboratory, a process I'll describe in detail in Chapter 10. Only when I am armed with a precise description of the problem can I understand it; only when I understand it can I prescribe proper therapy.

Therefore, when seeking help for your sleeping problem, you'll serve yourself and your physician better by being as specific and informative as you can be. Your thoughtful and carefully considered answers to the questions in the previous chapter are a good place to start. And if you do need to see a doctor for your sleeping disorder, take your responses to these questions with you to your appointment—you'll remember significant details when you have a written record with you.

MEDICAL CAUSES OF INSOMNIA

So intricate, so interconnected are our biological systems that I frequently feel a genuine sense of amazement that the body can work at all, let alone work so well for most people most of the time. However, the sheer number of things that can go physically wrong is also astounding, and it should come as no surprise that disruptions in virtually any body system can result in disturbed sleep. The following pages will offer an overview of some organic conditions that are potential sources of sleeping problems. You may recognize some of the symptoms as your own. But I must caution you about the difficulty of diagnosing your own condition. A symptom—headache, for example—can arise from a spectrum of causes. In any case, I strongly urge you to discuss with a physician any symptoms you experience. Any clues you are able to provide may be just the piece of information needed to understand, and remedy, your situation.

Headache

To start at the top, headaches are one of the primary causes of sleep disturbance. Specifically, the culprits are vascular headaches—those that involve blood vessels—as opposed to tension headaches, which involve muscles and occur primarily during the day.

Migraine is a form of vascular headache, characterized by searing, throbbing pain. Usually a migraine seems to occur in the entire head, although occasionally it is confined to one side. Some victims perceive an aura or a visual disturbance that signals the imminent arrival of a migraine, which is often first felt in or near the eyes. Attacks can last for hours, even for a day or more. A sufferer may experience nausea and vomiting; so debilitating is an attack that one patient remarked that she actually looked forward to the third episode of vomiting because she knew her migraine would soon be over. Examination generally reveals no neurological signs; a physician may order X rays, brain scans, or an EEG to rule out organic disease. Prevention is usually the best approach, as unfortunately there is little relief available once a migraine attack begins. Prevention may be achieved with medication such propranolol (marketed as Inderal) or methysergide (marketed as Sansert). The acute attack may be treated with ergot derivatives, or with mild analgesics such as aspirin or stronger analgesics such as codeine.

It should be remembered that these strong analgesics have addictive potential, and should be used with great care, if at all, in people with a history of substance abuse.

Headache is also a symptom of hypertension, a condition in which blood is forced through arteries at higher than normal rates of pressure. Essential hypertension—the most common form of high blood pressure—is somewhat mysterious, arising from no perceptible cause, whereas secondary hypertension is the result of some other medical condition, such as renal artery stenosis (narrowed arteries of the kidneys). Dietary approaches, including limited sodium intake, can help. A number of medications are available today that can control essential hypertension; the secondary variety may require drugs, surgery, or other therapies, depending on its cause.

Other types of headaches include the "cluster" (or histamine) headaches: severe, one-sided headaches that seem to switch on and off during sleep but may last for hours. Headaches may also be caused by infection, alcoholism, uremia (a condition in which toxins build up in the blood), and poisoning by carbon monoxide or other chemicals. Some materials used in arts and crafts, such as lead-based paints or dyes, may produce headache, especially when used in confined environments for extended periods of time. If you have headaches that keep you awake at night, be sure to discuss with your physician any hobbies or activities, including drinking, that might be contributing to your problem.

Generally victims report a family history of headaches, which are more likely to occur in women. The physiological changes brought about by the onset of the Rapid Eye Movement (REM) period of sleep seem to aggravate headaches.

Other Central Nervous System Disorders

Alzheimer's disease, epilepsy, and degenerative conditions including Parkinson's disease and multiple sclerosis can lead to insomnia, as can brain tumors or injuries and any of the many forms of brain infection collectively known as encephalitis. Excessive sleepiness may be the result of increased intracranial pressure, a collection of blood between membranes of the brain due to a rupture in a blood vessel; syphilis attacking the central nervous system; or hydrocephalus, a condition resulting from accumulated fluid in the brain.

Heart Trouble

Sleep can cause changes in the circulatory system, such as lowered heart rate and blood pressure levels, which may precipitate or aggravate stroke, heart attack, arrhythmias (irregular heart rhythms), and other cardiac conditions. Conversely, some types of heart disease may themselves lead to changes in sleep patterns.

Right ventricular failure (RVF) is a form of congestive heart failure, a syndrome in which the heart is unable to move the blood efficiently or normally through its chambers. As a result fluids build up and cause congestion in the blood vessels and the lungs. The condition is specifically described as either right or left ventricular failure, depending on which of the lower chambers of the heart is involved. Patients with RVF are often told to rest in bed to alleviate edema, the swelling of the ankles that results from the accumulation of fluids. As a consequence of this drainage, however, the patient feels the need to urinate frequently. The increased number of nightly trips to the bathroom can disrupt sleep and prevent the patient from enjoying a restful night.

Left ventricular failure (LVF) often causes acute pulmonary edema, or sudden accumulation of fluid in the lungs. Victims experience difficulty in breathing and anxiety associated with a sense of suffocation. Frequently people with this condition sleep—not too comfortably—in chairs. Because of the disruptions in their breathing, they will often awaken at night and try to find some kind of relief, either by opening a window or by going for a walk "to get some fresh air." Relief is often obtained through the judicious use of the class of drugs called diuretics, or "water pills," which increase the excretion of liquids. Again, however, the increased frequency of bathroom visits can affect sleep.

In atherosclerosis, often called hardening of the arteries, fatty substances called lipids accumulate in the artery walls, especially those of the heart, brain, and kidneys, where they turn to plaque and cause the artery to stiffen. The circulation then becomes sluggish, and insufficient oxygen is carried to the different parts of the body. The heart disease that results causes nearly one of every three deaths in the United States. In the earlier stages of the disease the brain, sensing it is being deprived of oxygen, emits a distress signal. The heart and lungs then begin working harder to step up the brain's oxygen supply, and the increased cardiopulmonary activity often results in fragmented sleep.

Angina is the choking or suffocating pain that arises when the myocardium, the thick central muscle of the heart, is deprived of oxygen, usually as a result of exertion or excitement. Some experts think that sleep-disrupting anginal attacks may be triggered by the physiologic changes of the REM stage, perhaps even by the emotional content of the dreams that occur during that part of the sleep cycle (see page 86).

Asthma

Asthma frequently attacks at night, causing victims to awaken with wheezing, coughing, and shortness of breath. A combination of circadian rhythms, each reaching its respective high or low point, is thought by many researchers to trigger these nocturnal attacks. Other sleep factors, including the horizontal position and the physiologic changes that accompany the REM sleep phase, may also play a role. Inhaled drugs called bronchodilators can widen bronchial passages and quickly alleviate the symptoms. Long-lasting medications are now being marketed which are designed to reach their peak of therapeutic activity during the early hours of the morning, when the risk of an asthma attack seems to be the greatest.

Chronic Obstructive Pulmonary Disease (COPD)

COPD is a general name for several conditions that prevent normal breathing and interrupt sleep. These conditions include emphysema, chronic bronchitis, and abnormally developed airways. Usually the symptoms—difficulty breathing on exertion, coughing, wheezing, and frequent respiratory infections—begin to appear in middle age, although the disease itself may be present for years before symptoms develop. Often the first sign is a mild "smoker's cough." Usually COPD is not curable, but treatment can relieve symptoms and control the dangerous, and sometimes fatal, exacerbations of the disease. Therapy depends on the exact nature of the illness and may involve drugs, inhalation therapy, exercise, and supportive therapy.

Sleep Apnea

Apnea is the disordered breathing that arises during failure of the autonomic nervous system that controls the lungs. The subsequent lack of oxygen sets off various alarm systems in the brain, which then activates a number of mechanisms to alleviate the problem; for example, your body might shift position in an effort to breathe more easily. If these lesser measures fail, your brain may "order" you to wake up quickly so that you can make a conscious effort to breathe. Sometimes snoring can also trigger an apneic attack.

In serious cases, sleep apnea can result in the accumulation of acids in the blood. Furthermore, small arterial branches may constrict, resulting in pulmonary arterial hypertension. In more severe cases sleep apnea increases the risk of stroke, ischemia (insufficient blood supply to the heart muscles or brain), and even death, due to the reduction of oxygen in the blood and the subsequent effects on blood flow from the heart. A more detailed discussion of sleep apnea as a specific type of sleep disorder appears in Chapters 5 and 6.

Other Respiratory Changes

Changes in the rate of breathing and the amount of inhaled gas, retention of lung secretions due to reduced clearance of fluids in the lung, and changes in the muscle tone of the upper airways all affect one's ability to sleep. Fortunately, these changes are insignificant in normal people, but as we have seen, they can have severe ramifications in those with one of the respiratory illnesses described above.

Ulcers

Ulcers—more precisely, peptic ulcers—are lesions that occur in the esophagus (the "food tube"), the stomach, or the duodenum (the first part of the small intestine); they attack as many as one out of seven people in this country. Gastric ulcer refers to an ulcer that occurs specifically in the lesser curvature of the stomach lining. Recent statistics show that, despite the earlier image of the typical ulcer victim as a hard-driven man, women are as prone to ulcers as men.

Ulcers result from a disruption in the normal balance between the system that secretes stomach acid and the system that protects the mucous membrane lining the stomach. The disruption, which increases secretion of stomach acid, occurs as a result of diet, stress, or other illness. In normal people the amount of acid secreted during sleep is lower than during the day. However, in ulcer patients it can be as much as three to twenty times higher. Some drugs, including aspirin, may increase the risk of developing ulcers. Fortunately, most ulcers can be treated easily and quickly with a number of effective drugs such as cimetidine (brand name: Tagamet). In many cases relief occurs virtually overnight, and healing takes place within about eight weeks, although the patient is always at risk that ulcers will recur.

Heartburn

Heartburn (or gastroesophageal reflux) arises from failure of the mechanisms designed to prevent the acidic contents of the stomach from passing back into the esophagus, a process known as reflux. The esophagus, lacking the protective lining found in the stomach, is sensitive to acid, which accounts for the burning sensation. If the stomach contents back up into the mouth, a sour taste is noticed. Other symptoms include coughing, choking, or a feeling of respiratory discomfort. Reflux is unpleasant but not usually serious, although in some cases the fluid may be breathed into the lungs and lead to aspiration pneumonia.

Some experts suggest that people who find their sleep disrupted by gastroesophageal reflux should try to eat their evening meal as early as possible, so that food has more time to be digested and to pass into the small intestine. Knowing, for example, that a heavy, calorie-rich, high-fat meal may take five hours or more to pass out of the stomach may help you plan your menu as well as your bedtime. Other management techniques include raising the head of the bed by six inches and avoiding substances such as coffee, alcohol, chocolate, and fats, which stimulate acid secretion. Smoking cessation can help, since smoking has been shown to weaken the esophageal sphincter which closes off the entrance to the stomach. Antacids and other drugs may also provide relief.

Bowel Disorders

Such conditions as enteritis, colitis, and irritable bowel syndrome may disrupt regularity of bowel action. Victims may awaken frequently, feeling an urgent need to visit the bathroom. There is no specific therapy for enteritis, although certain drugs may help relieve cramps and diarrhea. Even surgery will only alleviate, not cure, the condition. Treatment for colitis depends on the severity of the disease and ranges from diet, relaxation therapy, and some types of drugs to hospitalization for corticosteroid therapy or surgery in extreme cases. Irritable bowel syndrome, also known as spastic colon, is a psychological reaction to stress, not an organic illness. Recommended treatment usually involves psychological counseling and regulation of physical activity and diet; some types of drugs may relieve specific symptoms. Depression is often a factor in this syndrome and must be dealt with appropriately.

Pain and Trauma

Generally the forms of insomnia associated with disorders of the muscles, joints, and bones are reactions to pain, inflammation, and swelling. And obviously, a person whose broken arm is encased in a cast is likely to experience some trouble sleeping in normal positions. Similarly, amateur athletes who overextend themselves on the ski slopes or the racquetball court may find it hard to get an uninterrupted night's sleep. In such cases the insomnia is directly related to the trauma and will pass as the condition improves. Other conditions, such as "frozen shoulder," may disturb sleep, but treatment usually involves drugs to reduce pain, not specifically to induce sleep.

Arthritis

This painful condition can cause a form of insomnia by preventing the patient from falling asleep promptly. Although arthritis and other degenerative disorders such as spondylosis do not generally disturb sleep, many victims notice pain and stiffness on waking, either during the night or in the morning, which may be one of the effects of circadian patterns during sleep. Some arthritics report feeling fatigued in the afternoons. Often, occasional complete bed rest is prescribed; anti-inflammatory drugs usually help if symptoms recur.

Other Physical Causes of Insomnia

As I suggested earlier, our sleep patterns are inherited to a large degree. One study found that nearly half of the children of parents with sleep problems also reported difficulty sleeping; when one of the parents had the problem, so did almost 30 percent of their offspring, whereas only 18 percent of the children of parents with no insomnia had a sleep disturbance. Obviously, the only preventive therapy for genetic insomnia is to pick the right set of parents.

Hospital patients have dozens of reasons for experiencing insomnia. The trauma of institutionalization—unfamiliar surroundings, strange schedules, the presence of strangers, uncomfortable bedclothes—can cause all sorts of emotional and mental stress. Surgical procedures or drug therapies, while curing some problems, can disrupt other body cycles and cause irregular sleep patterns. Of course, the mere presence of the illness that required hospitalization in the first place can cause sleep disturbance. Patients in intensive care may be awakened dozens of times during the course of a day; their bodies may thus be unable to generate the full supply of hormones responsible for healing body tissues which are normally released during the various sleep stages.

Disruptions in the functioning of the endocrine and metabolic systems, such as diabetes, can also produce insomnia. Hyperthyroidism—overactivity of the thyroid, a gland, which is responsible for a number of metabolic functions including protein synthesis and oxygen consumption—lists insomnia as one of its many symptoms. Any number of prescription medications can create disruptions in sleep patterns. The use of birth control pills may produce nighttime awakenings in women, and the hormonal fluctuations of the menstrual cycle may also disrupt sleep. And in some cases a man's nocturnal erections can be painful enough to disturb his sleep.

Any condition that produces itching, rashes, or other skin problems, such as the peeling following sunburn, can reduce the ability to sleep and must be treated in the appropriate manner. Unhygienic conditions may also contribute to sleeping problems. Bedbugs, for example, while not common, are with us even in this modern age. Corticosteroid lotions will help relieve symptoms, while frequent laundering of bedclothes or purchase of a new mattress will encourage the little creatures to seek a home elsewhere.

Similarly, especially in warmer regions of the country, insufficient window screens may admit flies and mosquitoes which in turn can disturb sleep. One effective mosquito repellent is reported to be a machine that produces a startlingly accurate version of the love call of the male mosquito. Female mosquitoes—the only ones who seek and suck blood—are much more intent on feeding than they are on lovemaking and tend to stay away from any area in which they think a horny male is on the prowl. For those of us whose homes are not equipped with this device, some judicious repair of window screens or the use of netting or commercial repellents may be indicated.

LIFESTYLE-RELATED CAUSES OF INSOMNIA

We've seen how the way we function emotionally and physically has much to do with the way we sleep. Another set of factors concerns the way in which we choose to conduct our lives on a day-by-day, even a minute-by-minute, basis. These factors are in a very real sense within our control to a greater extent than most of the ones we've discussed up to this point. They involve our choices of living environment, career, and habits of work, rest, and play. By focusing on them in some detail, you may discover things you are doing to yourself that are contributing to, or actually causing, your sleep disorder.

Living Environment

Our living accommodations can have a tremendous influence on the way we sleep. Those who live in capacious mansions, for example, have the luxury of large bedrooms, isolated from the rest of the house and well insulated from light, noise, and other disturbances, including neighbors. Most of us, however, make do with smaller abodes or apartments, where the foibles of other members of the family or of neighbors all too often intrude unbidden on our sleeping space.

Sound can be a particularly difficult problem. Science has shown that any sound over 70 decibels—slightly louder than ordinary conversation—stimulates the nervous system. In the case of sudden or prolonged sounds, the blood pressure increases and there is a reduction in the supply of blood to the heart. At higher levels the heart begins to race, muscles in the chest contract, and the pupils dilate. Thus the sounds of food blenders (90 decibels) or passing motorcycles (120 decibels) can penetrate our sleep and cause us to awaken, eyes wide open and hearts beating furiously. Settling down again can take a good ten minutes or more.

The thin walls resulting from inexpensive construction techniques can plague homeowners and apartment-dwellers alike. Inadequate curtains or shades can admit too much light. Clutter can make some people uncomfortable. Even creaking floorboards may prevent the onset of sleep. A noisy television or stereo can mean hours of troubled rest for the hapless occupant of the adjoining room. One friend of mine knew that he would suffer early-morning insomnia exactly twice a week: on trash-collection days, when his neighbor's two Labrador retrievers would noisily announce the arrival of the garbage truck.

Economic reality forces many people to compromise on the allotment of space in their homes. The number of children may increase, for example, while the number of bedrooms remains constant. Parents who bring a baby's crib into their room may find that the child's slightest sniffle or whimper is enough to keep two adults awake for hours. Children who share bedrooms may find that one sibling's nocturnal arousals—bed-wetting or sleep-walking, for example—interrupt the sleep of all. Snuggling together in bed is one chief attraction of cohabitation, but the partner of a snorer who has no other sleeping space may find that pleasure somewhat diminished. Even the purchase of lesser-quality mattresses and pillows may contribute to nighttime discomfort.

Family tensions militate against adequate sleep. Couples who argue may be unable to disguise their battles from the children upstairs or down the hall and may thus fail to shield them from the emotional fallout. Unresolved arguments or ongoing conflicts over anything from schoolwork to social life to household responsibilities also take their toll at night. In many cases family counseling can serve to ease these tensions; often, too, simple constructive discussions can do much to air differences and provide solutions. If you or someone in your family is having trouble sleeping, a long, thoughtful look at your family's group dynamics might reveal that the cause of the problem at night lies in your interactions during the day.

Job-Related Stress

To some degree, this form of anxiety is virtually ubiquitous in our society. Many families find that there is never enough money to meet present demands while planning for future desires. Just when we think we've overcome one financial crisis, one of the kids flushes his socks down the toilet and the plumber presents us with a whopping repair bill. Or, more seriously, illness will strike, depleting a family's meager reserves. Sometimes a worker holds two jobs, or both partners work out of financial necessity, not by choice. The tensions that arise from an employee's desire to perform well and to please bosses and co-workers—and family members—sometimes intermingle with feelings of boredom or career dissatisfaction, leading to a frequent, if not constant, desire to "chuck it all."

In addition, many people "take their jobs to bed" with them when they turn in. Perhaps you lie awake for half an hour or so, mentally running down your calendar of appointments for the following day. Perhaps you rehearse your sales presentation or outline the steps you need to take to complete a project. You may replay scenes of confrontation over and over, working yourself up into a state of rage over some insult, real or imagined. You may continually rewrite past scenes so that—in your head, at least—you succeed where before you failed, or so that you deliver just the right remark at just the right opportunity. You may worry about a promotion, a layoff, a shift in responsibilities, or the arrival of a new employee. Any of these situations can trigger a troubled night's sleep.

The solution, of course, depends on the actual situation. Some may find that a discussion with their employer or co-workers will settle an issue or create harmony. Others may need to reshuffle their responsibilities or work load. Occasionally just asking for help can work wonders. A patient I'll call Lisa—a shy but capable woman in her forties—was working ten- and twelve-hour days just to keep up with her responsibilities as print production manager for a small publishing company. Often she found herself taking work home in the evening, hoping to catch up. Consequently she spent less and less time with her children, thus further losing out on the pleasures of her home life. She was reluctant to mention the situation to her boss, fearing that he would find her incapable of handling her duties and dismiss her. The stress eventually manifested itself as a problem in dropping off to sleep. Through role-playing we were able to rehearse a meeting with her boss. In Lisa's case the clinical setting and the participation of a professional counselor helped her find new ways of approaching the problem and relieved her of the need to ruminate over the situation at bedtime. Normal sleep returned when she at last was able to confront her employer, who agreed to hire a part-time assistant.

Shift Work

Working different shifts at odd hours is a notorious disrupter of sleep. In the United States, over 13 million people—roughly 20 percent of the work force—work either full-time or part-time shifts in the evening or at night. A surprising variety of people work hours other than the standard nine to five: actors, disk jockeys, journalists, and broadcasters; waiters, cooks, and bakers; truckers, taxi drivers, and train engineers; police, fire fighters, and security guards; air-traffic controllers, pilots, and cabin crews; computer programmers, communications workers, and telephone operators; doctors, residents, nurses, and medical students; construction crews and road repair teams; soldiers and sailors; athletes, salesclerks, students, maintenance personnel, and turnpike toll takers.

The statistical profile of shift workers is revealing. In one study, shift workers were twice as likely as day workers to report trouble sleeping; one plant's personnel registered a rate of sleep difficulty of 76 percent. Another study reported that half of all shift workers fell asleep on the job at least once a week. Of course, on-the-job napping can pose a threat not only to workers and colleagues but to the public as a whole, as in the case of security guards, transportation workers, and plant operators.

The nuclear accidents at Chernobyl and Three Mile Island were in part the consequence of decisions made by sleepy shift workers. One study also found that 15 percent of the shift workers reported falling asleep while behind the wheel of a car at least once every three months. These drowsy drivers are a hazard to themselves and everyone else on the road.

The problem is compounded on weekends when, naturally, these workers try to adopt a schedule that permits them to interact socially with family and friends, most of whom enjoy a nine-to-five work day.

The sleep disruptions caused by shift work have an impact on productivity as well. People who follow unusual work schedules average only 5.6 hours of sleep a day. Besides being less alert on the job, they are prone to a number of disorders, especially digestive ailments, because the rhythms that control the release of enzymes, hormones, and digestive acids have been thrown off. On average, shift workers are absent from their jobs an additional five days a year compared with others in the labor force—not because of illness but because of the effects of fatigue. The cost of such absenteeism must be reckoned in the billions of dollars. To compensate for their sleep difficulties, shift workers are liable to nap more, drink more caffeine, use over-the-counter stimulants, consume more alcohol, and rely on hypnotic drugs to induce sleep. At one plant two out of every three shift workers used alcohol at bedtime at least once a week, and 12 percent used sleeping pills at the same frequency.

As should be clear, one key problem in trying to adjust to shift work is the constant battle between the demands of the job and the demands of the body. Workers who punch in at midnight and try to sleep during the day are attempting to suppress their body's natural clock, ignoring a million years of evolutionary programming in order to conform to a man-made time structure. They must learn to ignore the light–dark cycle—the prime time cue that drives the internal clocks of thousands of species. What's more, they lack the reinforcement of time cues provided by society at large: watching the seven o'clock evening news broadcasts, taking meals at regular hours, and so on. Small wonder that they must pay a price in increased fatigue, sleepiness, illness, absenteeism, and disruption in their family and social lives.

Some enlightened employers, sensitive to the demands of the circadian cycle, attempt to correct the problem by rotating shifts to allow workers' bodies to catch up with themselves. Following this strategy, a coal company in the Midwest reported a 10 percent increase in productivity after adopting a schedule that rotates shifts every four weeks and gives workers a seven-day break before they begin the new shift. A number of major corporations, including Exxon and Dow Chemical, also give workers a few days off between shift changes. After the Philadelphia Police Department began a program to reduce shift changes, it reported a 40 percent decline in job-related traffic accidents and a 50 percent drop in complaints of daytime fatigue. In addition, 25 percent fewer officers said they slept poorly.

In fact, among shift workers in general, 27 percent of men and 16 percent of women now participate in rotating shift schedules. A typical twenty-eight-day plan has workers take a day shift for seven days or so. After a number of days off—anywhere from one to four—the worker takes the night shift for another week, then moves to the evening shift following another few days off. Unfortunately, say the experts, such a plan rotates in the wrong direction. One study found that the most satisfied shift workers were those whose schedules rotated forward—day–evening–night—and who also changed shifts in ten-day, rather than seven-day, cycles.

Obviously many people who work shifts are not given the luxury of designing optimum work schedules for themselves. But if you suspect your sleep difficulty stems from such a work arrangement, there may be channels through which you can discuss the problem with co-workers, union representatives, or management. Becoming aware of the improvements in worker attitude, productivity, and health that can result from recognizing our circadian natures may convince those who control work schedules that adjustments can be made to benefit everyone concerned.

Use of Chemicals and Stimulants

Alcohol can have a striking impact on our sleep patterns. The alcoholic nightcap is perhaps one of the most deeply ingrained habits in many people's lives. Yet alcohol harms sleep by suppressing the REM, or dream, phase of sleep. REM "rebounds" later in the night, after the alcohol has been absorbed, often resulting in troubling dreams. Recently some experts have come to believe that less than one shot—one ounce—of liquor taken within an hour or so of bedtime can disturb sleep patterns, making sleep light, unsettled, and unrefreshing.

Caffeine This is sometimes deliberately consumed by people in an effort to keep themselves stimulated and awake. Unfortunately, many of us consume much more than we need to achieve this effect, and we continue to ingest it right up until bedtime. Many patients tell me they "only drink three cups of coffee a day," then casually mention that the cup they use is a 16-ounce mug! If they have a Coke or a chocolate bar at lunch, they may be ingesting nearly 1,500 milligrams of caffeine a day—the equivalent of ten six-ounce cups. (Caffeine is an element not only in coffee, cola, and chocolate, but in tea, other soft drinks, including Dr Pepper and Mountain Dew, and numerous over-the-counter medications, including Anacin, Dristan, Empirin, Excedrin, Midol, and Vanquish.)

Some experts, although they lack hard proof, believe that caffeine may act to reset our body's natural time clock. If this turns out to be true, we may be disrupting our internal rhythms by forcing them to recycle back to "go" every time we drink a cup of coffee. As a rule, try to curtail all use of caffeine after 6:00 P.M. If you have a persistent problem falling asleep, you might try to do without caffeine completely.

Nicotine This is the drug contained in cigarette smoke. It can affect sleep, surprisingly, to an even greater degree than caffeine. Compared with nonsmokers, smokers take a longer time falling asleep—up to fourteen minutes more, in one study—and are awake during the night nearly twenty minutes longer. In addition, smoking can rob the blood of oxygen, making apnea worse and further reducing the flow of oxygen to the brain. Sleep often improves dramatically in smokers who quit: investigators have found that the amount of time awake during the night decreased nearly 50 percent in two-pack-a-day smokers who quit. There are, of course, numerous other health benefits to quitting.

Your physician can work with you to plan the smoking-cessation strategy that will work best in your case.

Marijuana This drug often induces a heavy sleepy feeling in users; their eyelids droop and they fall into a state of lethargy. Often their sleep is shallow and fragmented, and they wake in the morning feeling fatigued and depressed.

Cocaine Whether injected, sniffed, or smoked, cocaine produces feelings of stimulation, alertness, and euphoria, much the same as high doses of amphetamines. Because it is short-acting, users frequently give themselves numerous doses, through either injection or inhalation. Toxic effects include abnormal heartbeats, hypertension, muscle-twitching, dilation of the pupils, extreme nervousness, and hallucinations. Not surprisingly, sleeplessness is another side effect.

Other lifestyle factors Diet can affect sleep. I mentioned the role that heavy, fatty foods can play in aggravating heartburn. Some nutritionists also believe that eating a sweet snack at bedtime may cause a rush of sleep-disturbing energy; other experts, it should be noted, feel that ingesting carbohydrates actually causes sleepiness.

For some people, reading or watching TV before bedtime provides more stimulation than is appropriate at this time of night. Also, if you exercise late in the evening, you may be stirring up your bodily systems and making it difficult for them to settle down come bedtime. Exercise raises the body temperature, which may prevent the onset of sleep. The stimulation of aggressive competition, such as a game of tennis with the number-one seeded player in your office intramural tournament, can take a while to pass from your system. Don't stop exercising, but try to move the exercise to a point no later than two to four hours before you turn in.

Sexual activity does not count as late-night exercise, of course. Many people are aware of the sleep-inducing side effects of normal, healthy intercourse at bedtime. However, studies have shown that men are actually more likely than women to fall asleep after sex. What's more, men's sleep stages after sex show no differences from those on nights without sexual activity.

Women, on the other hand, experience less deep sleep following sex, spending more time in lighter sleep. One interpretation is that women are less likely than their male partners to feel sexually satisfied; their bodily systems have been fired up but have not been allowed to relax through the release that orgasm provides. In fact, 60 to 70 percent of women who complain of insomnia also report a high degree of sexual frustration.

A change in routine or lifestyle can also take some time to get used to. People entering retirement frequently experience disturbed sleep for up to three weeks until they adopt a new pattern, one compatible with their new situation. "Old-age boredom" can be a hidden cause of insomnia. Sometimes people become involved in a project, hobby, or other activity that produces an erratic sleep schedule. If bedtime varies by two or three hours a night, the circadian cycle may be disrupted and need to be reset. I have learned to recognize that patients who describe themselves as "night owls" may in fact be suffering from the type of insomnia known as delayed sleep phase syndrome, in which they find it difficult to fall asleep at a normal hour and thus have difficulty waking in the morning.

JET LAG

There is an insidious form of sleep disturbance, quite definitely a product of lifestyle, which has been clinically recognized only within the last decade or so. This sleeping disorder attacks millions of people each year, yet most of them are unaware that the disease is treatable—perhaps even preventable. It goes by the descriptive, if somewhat unscientific, name of jet lag.

Years ago, when I first heard complaints about this form of travel sickness, I tended to dismiss the symptoms as being largely psychosomatic—the airborne equivalent of mild *mal de mer*. Then I flew to Europe to attend a medical convention and realized firsthand what all the talk was about, not due to the learned talks delivered by my colleagues but because of the debilitating case of jet lag I suffered.

Jet lag is the disruption of the body's circadian rhythms, brought about by rapid travel to another time zone. And no wonder these cycles go haywire: virtually every physiological and environmental clue we use to reset our internal clocks changes the moment our feet touch the ground in a new part of the world.

When we travel from New York to London, we may leave, say, at eight o'clock in the morning, local time. The flight may take only about seven hours, meaning we land at three in the afternoon—again, our own personal local time. But we have crossed five time zones and landed in a strange new world where the inhabitants live five hours in the future. We have thus "lost" five hours of our lives. We don't panic, of course, because we know we'll get them back when we return to New York. But, as I discovered, the effects of this form of time travel may linger with us for weeks.

It should not be surprising that the body's natural time clock—the light–dark cycle—is the first system to break down. In our example, we may leave New York early on a bright sunny morning and arrive in damp, foggy London at eight o'clock *in the evening* London time. If you count time in the air as a form of suspended animation, we have essentially pushed our clocks forward by twelve hours. (Compare this to daylight saving time, which involves only one hour.) In the blink of an eye—well, almost—we have turned day into night. Small wonder the light–dark cycle goes on red alert, trying to figure out just what is happening and how to cope with it.

But other time cues are in turmoil as well. Odds are we were up the night before, packing frantically or making last-minute plans. Possibly our sleep was disrupted by excitement about the trip. We rose early, skipping breakfast to be sure we made it to the airport in time. After a less-than-adequate meal on the plane we dozed fitfully in an unusual (some would say impossible) position. Later in the flight we might have eaten another meal, accompanied by an alcoholic drink or two. On landing we get settled in the hotel and go immediately to dinner, since by then it may be ten or eleven o'clock local time. Then, at perhaps two in the morning, we turn in for a good night's sleep.

What's wrong with this picture? Everything. The day of our flight begins after a troubled night. Our diet is different, in composition as well as in time of consumption. We take a nap—perhaps something we almost never do. We arrive in darkness and rush around to fulfill our need for shelter and food, both of which, when found, may be unfamiliar if not downright strange. Once those needs are satisfied, our bodies try their best to accommodate our demand that they sleep.

Obviously our internal time clock is at odds with our new reality. Everything—body temperature, adrenaline secretion, alertness and performance levels, circulating brain chemicals—has become desynchronized. As a result our sleep can be severely disturbed, thus setting in motion another vicious circle: without adequate sleep, our immunity is lower; our resistance is down. We may become ill or fatigued, resulting in further physiological breakdown, causing a worsening of sleep disturbance. The rest of the trip can be, as you may well know from your own experience, a disaster. It may take as long as one full day per time zone traveled to adjust to local conditions. One survey found that daytime sleepiness and fatigue affect 90 percent of jet lag victims, while inability to sleep at night is found in 78 percent. Predictably, the elderly are more prone to jet lag, perhaps because their daily cycles may already be in some state of deterioration.

Jet lag seems to affect people more after a trip from west to east, such as the example I've given, than after a trip from east to west—for example, from Los Angeles to Japan. When you head east, your day grows shorter; heading west, however, your day grows longer and poses a lesser threat to your normal biological cycle.

The effects of jet lag pose a very real danger to our ability to perform. Take, for example, the case of John Foster Dulles, Secretary of State under Eisenhower. In the 1950s Dulles flew to Egypt and immediately entered into negotiations for a treaty concerning the construction of the Aswan High Dam. The United States lost the contract to the Soviets, however, and political observers note that the loss led to years of Soviet influence in the region. Dulles later stated that jet lag was a major factor in his failure to secure the Aswan contract, and he advised all U.S. diplomats to avoid conducting important meetings so soon after long-distance travel. More recently, U.S. Olympic diver Greg Louganis blamed jet lag for causing him to hit his head on a diving platform during the 1979 trials in Moscow. Traveling, he said, had diminished his coordination and thrown off his timing.

There are a number of techniques you can use to forestall, or at least minimize, the consequences of jet lag. If I had known about some of them before that medical convention, I might have been able to stay awake through the presentations and retain some of what I heard.

The first item on the agenda is—the agenda. The basic rule here is to *plan your schedule* so as to defeat the forces that may disrupt your circadian timing. If you will be traveling for only a short time—say a two-day business trip—you may be better off doing nothing rather than trying to adjust your schedule dramatically. It's better to try to live on your local time to the extent possible for the duration of your stay. However, if you are planning a month-long romp with a Eurailpass, action is called for. Here are ten suggestions for minimizing the impact of jet lag.

1. Start early

A few days before you leave home, begin to move toward the time frame that governs life in the part of the world you'll be visiting. If possible, gradually adjust your sleep schedule by rising earlier (when traveling east) or later (when traveling west). Make similar modifications in your eating schedule. (Naturally, if you find it difficult to do so, or if your sleeping pattern undergoes a change for the worse, stop.)

2. Don't push

Plan your packing ahead of time. Jot down items you want to bring and assemble them over the course of a few days or a week, so you're not frantically scrambling to collect them two hours before your flight. Confirm your plans several days in advance to avoid last-minute surprises. Don't crowd your calendar on the day (and night) before your departure. Avoid farewell celebrations, heavy meals, and alcoholic drinks. Just make your departure quietly, without fanfare.

3. Enjoy your flight

Make things easy on yourself. Dress comfortably; get to the airport in plenty of time; eat a light meal; read the paper. Once on board, avail yourself of the many diversions. Browse through one of the magazines you've never bothered to buy. Spring for the earphones and watch the movie. Talk with your traveling companion or seatmates. Get out of your seat at least once an hour to stretch or to freshen up.

4. Don't work!
If it's a business trip, keep your laptop computer stashed under your seat. Don't revise the text of your speech or review your notes.

5. Keep it light
Eat sparingly during the flight. Take no more than one alcoholic drink, if any. Don't smoke, or, if that is impossible on longer flights, try keeping to a maximum of one cigarette every two hours. Try leaving your cigarettes in your (checked) luggage, if you can. Drink decaffeinated coffee, or ask for orange or tomato juice instead.

6. Plan ahead I
Consider the day of the flight a travel day only. Try to schedule your arrival for late in the day, as close as possible to bedtime back home. This way you won't be so tempted to "see the town" before you turn in.

7. Ease into travel
Don't crowd your first full day with constant activities. Plan a leisurely rise, enjoy the morning meal, and set out when you feel ready. Keep activities light and nonstrenuous. Stroll through a village; don't climb an Alp.

8. Eat easy
See below for more details about diet.

9. Rest easy
To the extent possible, re-create your back-home bedtime ritual. Follow the same teeth-brushing, pillow-fluffing, sheep-counting routine you use at home. Bring relaxing reading. If you're worried about missing a wake-up call, bring your own trusty alarm clock.

10. Plan ahead II
Allow at least one day—two is better—to readjust upon your return. Try to avoid coming back to a desk full of work and piled-up assignments. Give yourself time to get back up to

speed: don't try to read all the accumulated mail in one day. Throw away nine-tenths of the newspapers that you missed.

Obviously, most of us seldom have so much control over our schedule that we can indulge ourselves with all the luxuries I've just outlined. But even if you adopt only three or four of these rules, you'll minimize the impact of travel and improve the quality of your rest.

Jet Lag and Diet

A number of diets have been designed that purport to provide relief for the symptoms of jet lag. Some are founded on the simple principle that intake of caffeine may serve to reset the circadian clock. However, such an effect has not yet been firmly demonstrated in humans. Thus, while jet lag diets are well intentioned, there is little evidence that they actually work and much controversy about their usefulness.

One dietary approach has been shown to be effective in U.S. military personnel who had to be in top form after a flight to Europe to participate in NATO war games. This plan, developed by a research laboratory in Illinois, recommends that you alternate between heavy meals ("feasts") and light ones ("fasts"), and between meals loaded with carbohydrates and those containing high amounts of protein.

Day 3 preflight (feast):	Breakfast:	Protein, high calorie
	Lunch:	Protein, high calorie
	Dinner:	Carbohydrate, high calorie
Day 2 preflight (fast):	Breakfast:	Low carbohydrate, low calorie
	Lunch:	Low carbohydrate, low calorie
	Dinner:	Low carbohydrate, low calorie
Day 1 preflight (feast):	Same as Day 3, above	
Flight day (fast):	Small meals	
	Avoid carbohydrates and caffeine	

In flight:	Avoid heavy meals	
	Take high-protein breakfast as near to landing as possible	
	Have coffee before landing	
Arrival day:	Lunch:	Large, high-protein meal
	Dinner:	Ample, carbohydrate-rich meal

As you may know, foods containing carbohydrates are cereals, breads, fruits, and starchy vegetables such as potatoes, rice, and corn. Protein-rich foods include meat, eggs, and milk. Combinations such as rice and beans complement each other by providing what is known as complete protein.

While this approach may work for you, the most important thing, as always, is to use common sense. Obviously, a balanced diet is always important; too much of anything is unhealthy. Our natural tendency when traveling is to eat large, heavy meals in an effort to indulge ourselves in new experiences. If you suddenly flood your system with spicy, rich, or otherwise unusual foods, consumed on an erratic schedule, you may only aggravate the other symptoms of jet lag. Your sleeping pattern will be disrupted, not only for the time you are traveling but for days or weeks following your return.

Other Jet Lag Strategies

For more thorough management of jet lag, there's a form of therapy you should know about which involves manipulating our circadian light–dark cycle. Basically, the idea is to do all you can to convince your body that the sun is rising and setting at a different time. The trick is simply one of controlled exposure to light.

Exposure to light sets the biologic clock that controls a number of circadian cycles. One effect of light is that it suppresses the secretion of melatonin, which is a neurotransmitter that produces feelings of sleepiness and, in excess quantities, symptoms of depression. Through appropriate timing of our exposure to light we can control the release of melatonin. This in turn will help reduce the severity of jet lag—at least in our subjective assessment of its effects—although it may not actually cause objective improvements in our performance once we've landed.

If you wish to try this approach, and you plan to travel east in a week or so, make it a point to step outside for about fifteen minutes as soon as convenient after sunrise. Contrarily, if you're headed west, take a stroll in the afternoon. If the trip will be particularly long (for example, from Los Angeles to Paris), some experts advise that a few days before your trip you should avoid early exposure to the sun but seek early exposure after you've arrived. Bright artificial light can also work, but to be effective the light intensity (measured in units called lux) should be about 2,000 to 2,500 lux—less than that of natural daylight, which ranges from 10,000 to 100,000 lux, but about four times the level of ordinary indoor lighting. One airline is even considering installing bright lights on flights traveling east or west to help passengers adjust. (Light therapy has also been found to be effective in manipulating the sleep cycles of patients who suffer from advanced or delayed onset of sleep, and it could conceivably be used to help shift workers adjust to their unusual schedules.)

For severe cases of jet lag, some drug therapies may be helpful. The National Institute of Mental Health recommends the use of a short-acting benzodiazepine hypnotic such as triazolam over the course of a few nights when it's important to avoid transient insomnia. Also, some benefits have been seen in people who have taken oral doses of melatonin; research in this area, however, is really just beginning.

SUMMARY

As you can see, virtually any of our daily activities—eating, drinking, exercise, leisure, travel—can pose a threat to our sleep. Our American way of life, for all its virtues, has produced a culture—one flooded with electric light and throbbing with virtually round-the-clock stimulation—where people are sleeping less than at any time in history. This loss of sleep possesses a cumulative effect, a form of "sleep debt" which many of us never pay back. And as we've seen, the consequences can be deadly, not only for the sleep-deprived person but for others as well.

To understand the consequences of going without sleep, we must examine why we need to sleep in the first place. Even the experts can't agree on the answer to this question. But, as we'll see in the next chapter, by understanding the sleep process we gain insight into this mysterious aspect of our lives and into the consequences that may occur when we can't sleep.

3

The Importance
of Sleep

Years ago, as a resident in training, I endured—as had thousands of would-be physicians before me—the rigorous demands of medical education. Part of this ordeal included a seemingly endless string of sleepless days and nights as I crammed countless facts about anatomy, pharmacology, and diseases into my skull. Sometimes, hard on the heels of these intense eighteen- and twenty-four-hour study sessions, I would be called to the hospital wards to tend to the needs of patients or follow my instructors on their rounds. Looking back, I sometimes get the impression—an erroneous one, to be sure—that my years of medical school were uninterrupted by even the briefest period of sleep.

At certain moments during the roughest times, as I struggled, usually vainly, to keep my eyelids open and my head erect, the question formed in my increasingly foggy mind: why do I have to sleep?

Since then I have participated in dozens of conversations with colleagues, patients, and friends, in which the principal topic is sleep. Some hard-charging, deadline-driven types will complain that the need to sleep simply interferes with their lives and their work. Others bemoan their inability to pass a trouble-free night, one without disturbing dreams or mind-numbing wakefulness. Still others delight in their ability to drop off the minute their head hits the pillow and to sleep soundly until morning arrives.

Not once in any of these conversations, nor in any of the voluminous literature on the subject, have I encountered a satisfactory answer to my seemingly simple question.

Why do we sleep?

Why are our bodies designed so that we must spend a third of our lives—perhaps twenty-five years or more!—in the unconsciousness of sleep? And if sleep is so vital to our well-being, why does it sometimes hesitate to descend on us or refuse to linger long once it has arrived?

Today medical science has the ability to transplant living organs from one body to another. We dissolve kidney stones with sound waves, and with the help of a computer we peer into the living brain. In the future we will have a complete map of the human genetic structure and will use that map to predict, and ultimately to forestall, the consequences of an inherited tendency toward crippling diseases ranging from Alzheimer's to alcoholism. So far, however, science has not come up with a positive, or even an adequate, answer to my question. The truth is, no one knows for certain. Perhaps there is poetic justice in the fact that the purpose of this basic biological function, associated as it is with night, darkness, closed doors, and closed eyelids, should evade even the most diligent investigators.

For centuries writers, poets, and philosophers have pondered the mysteries and meaning of sleep. Aristotle, for example, proposed that sleep occurred when the "vapors" of the head cooled down at night. In the centuries since Aristotle, sleep was generally assumed to be a temporary and partial shutting down of mental and biological activity, just as a windmill ceases to operate when the wind dies down.

It now seems strange that until the middle of this century the tools of medical science, which had been brought to bear on virtually every aspect of bodily function, were applied only occasionally to the subject of sleep. Why did scientific investigators seem reluctant to probe too deeply into the subject? Perhaps they simply took sleep as a given, one of little intrinsic interest.

Or perhaps they focused on the waking hours because only during that time could they exercise any degree of control over the subjects under study. It may simply be that the proper tools were not available to make such research fruitful. Had the electroencephalograph (EEG) been at Aristotle's disposal, for example, he would have been able to observe the rapid changes in brain waves generated during sleep, and he would have realized that during this period the brain is anything but "cool."

In the early 1950s, sleep research began in earnest. Two researchers in Chicago began to investigate the slow rolling eye movements that accompany the onset of sleep and decided to track the movements throughout the night. They soon noticed a hitherto undescribed kind of eye movement—rapid and furious, compared to the slow movement they had set out to study. By associating such movements with distinctive brain waves recorded by electroencephalograph, they helped crystallize the notion that sleep, far from being a shutting down, was an active state, especially as far as the brain was concerned and especially during this period of rapid eye movement (REM).

In the intervening decades there has been more research on sleep—more discoveries, more data—than in the previous two millennia. Sleep research has benefited from the cross-fertilization provided by a multidisciplinary approach, one which combines research in brain chemistry and structure, body function, and mental processes. The results, while by no means complete, have brought about a new understanding of the mechanisms of sleep and the processes that disrupt it.

That sleep is important cannot be overstressed. As I have mentioned, it is now known, for example, that the nuclear power accidents at both Three Mile Island in Pennsylvania and Chernobyl in the Soviet Union, which occurred in the early hours of the morning, were at least partially the result of bad decisions made by night-shift workers, a group particularly prone to disruptions in their sleep cycles. One study found that some airline crashes can be attributed to faulty decisions made by pilots, for whom sleep disruption is an occupational hazard. And nearly everyone knows the awful feeling of dozing off, even for the slightest split second, behind the wheel of a car doing 55 (or more) miles an hour.

Although it is easy to list the things that can go wrong when we don't sleep—accidents, errors in judgment, illness—we are still left without an answer to the basic question: Why do we sleep?

THE BIOLOGICAL BASIS FOR SLEEP

Following are some of the theories that have been proposed to explain the existence and purpose of sleep. As you'll see from the counterarguments presented, no single theory supplies all the answers to our query.

Theory #1: "Sleep Provides Rest for the Brain."

Simple common sense would seem to dictate that we sleep in order to rest. Virtually all working machines, whether natural or man-made, demonstrate a need for rest. Obviously, you can't run your car's engine at full speed for weeks or even days without risking a breakdown. Similarly, for organic creatures, sleep seems to be a period of inactivity forced upon the biologic system in order to prevent its total collapse.

Even as they function in our waking hours, the muscles and organs of the body are given a chance to rest. Our eyelids, our lungs, even our hearts stop moving for a period of time, if only for a fraction of a second, between cycles. The weight lifter pauses after each bench press before moving on to the next one. Muscle growth apparently occurs not during the strain of lifting, which actually serves to break down tissue, but in the period of recovery that follows, during which tissue is rebuilt. But rest, as seen in these examples, simply means a period of inactivity that can be achieved without descending into complete unconsciousness. Our hearts beat over 2 billion times in the course of an average human life-span, yet they don't need to stop working for eight hours in order to function well for another sixteen. If our bodies demand rest—and obviously they do—why are we not able to attain it merely by sitting or lying immobile for a few minutes or a few hours each day? Why must we "take leave of our senses," surrendering control of our awareness, simply to attain the rest which other systems manage to achieve even as they continue to function?

Researchers attempting to answer this question focus their attention on the brain. In contrast to other parts of the body, the brain is not granted the luxury of complete rest. It continues to operate every moment of the day. The only time it can relax to any extent is when less input is being received from the outside. Sleep, it would seem, makes such a reduction in sensory activity possible and, in mammals at least, seems to permit some form of restitution for the brain. Perhaps, then, sleep simply provides the degree of "shutdown" necessary for cerebral rest to take place. However, as we'll see later, even this degree of rest can occur during only about 75 percent of the night, during those stages of sleep when dreaming does not take place.

The need for cerebral rest may therefore be one reason, perhaps even the main reason, why we sleep. But it does not account for all of the physical and mental processes that occur in the night.

Theory #2: "Sleep Is a Way of Conserving Energy."

This seems to be true for animals, including less advanced mammals, for whom sleep acts as an immobilizer. And it may have been true at one time in the evolutionary history of the human species. Tens of thousands of years ago, when our primitive ancestors spent every waking hour in a struggle against their environment, the simple need to eat and stay warm consumed their energy at a prodigious rate. These creatures might have needed an involuntary period of enforced rest in order to be at their peak for the inevitable struggle the following day.

In our somewhat more advanced culture, however, the fight for heat and food is somewhat less of an ordeal. We might kick and scream when our furnaces go on the blink, but usually the solution is as simple as calling a repairman. We aren't cursed with having to wait for lightning to strike in order to have our fires rekindled. And the search for a meal need be no more complicated than phoning for a pizza, or any more anxiety-provoking than hoping it arrives before it gets cold.

So many people lead sedentary lifestyles—sitting at desks during the day, "cocooning" in front of the TV at night—that they are virtually as physically inactive while awake as they are lying in bed. Thus sleep is now considered to be a more important energy-saving mechanism for animals than it is for us humans, who are able to obtain at least some rest while we are awake. Some scientists even suggest that energy conservation may now be only a minor function of human sleep.

What's more, the deep, restful sleep which may be thought of as "obligatory" for providing rest usually takes place during the first few hours of the night. Gradually this obligatory sleep gives way to the more "optional" level of sleep occupied by dreaming. In a sense, then, we do our required "sleep homework" when we first go to bed. We are then allowed to enjoy the dream-laden sleep which appears less necessary to our physical survival, but which, as we will see, may have a great deal to do with the emotional level of functioning that defines our very humanity.

Theory #3: "Sleep Recharges Our Batteries."

Again, this would appear to be common sense, a version of the law of conservation of energy. Or, put another way, for every action there must be a compensating reaction: if you expend two hours of energy, you must spend an hour in sleep to regain it. Such an interplay of forces, a kind of kinetic yin and yang, must surely be a governing biological principle.

Not so, apparently. People who have gone without sleep for up to 260 hours needed only 15 extra hours or so, spread over a few nights, to return to normal sleeping patterns. In other words, we don't really need an hour of sleep to make up for two hours of wakefulness.

Theory #4: "Sleep Promotes Tissue Growth."

It is true that during the first few hours of sleep the human pituitary gland releases large amounts of growth hormone. But the same hormone is also released during the day; it's just that the mechanisms controlling the release are different after night falls. In fact, growth hormone is not even released in significant amounts during sleep in most of us over the age of forty.

As the body gets older, the function of the growth hormone also changes; it serves more to slow down the degradation of our tissues than to actively promote growth and repair. At this stage of life, then, the hormone acts somewhat like the groundskeeper who maintains an existing garden rather than the landscaper who plans and plants one. Besides, if the function of sleep were merely to promote growth-hormone activity, then we humans would be virtually unique in that regard, since nocturnal release of growth hormone occurs in only a few animals. It does not, for example, take place in cats or rats.

Theory #5: "Sleep Triggers the Process of Tissue Repair."

Scientists have indeed observed that in humans cell division (and thus in a sense cell restitution) tends to reach its peak in the early-morning hours. It therefore would appear that cell division (technically known as mitosis) is caused by sleep. But this association is only coincidental. Mitosis takes place in a daily cycle, or circadian rhythm, which happens to reach its peak at the same time we sleep. Sleep does not govern this circadian rhythm, nor does it directly cause cell division to occur. Nor, for that matter, is mitosis likely to stop in people who are deprived of sleep. Moreover, cell "growth" may not actually occur at all, since cells are constantly dying off even as they are being replaced. We don't know enough about the rate of cell death during sleep to determine if there's a net gain in the number of cells by the time we rise and shine.

Other research seems to indicate that eating, not sleeping, triggers regeneration of tissue through protein metabolism—the process that breaks down protein and converts it to energy. Studies have shown that our rate of protein metabolism drops during sleep at night. However, if you awaken and eat a snack, your rate of protein turnover will remain constant. These results suggest that it is your intake of food that regulates tissue repair, not any intrinsic factor involved with sleep.

Theory #6: "Sleep Helps Fortify Us Against Disease."

This argument may have some merit. During the deepest stages of the sleep cycle, it appears that the immune system is strengthened in some ways. Whether this strengthening is triggered by sleep or occurs coincidentally during the nighttime hours is a subject for debate. However, such an immunological process may account for the weakened resistance to disease that is one consequence of insufficient sleep.

Also, people who are already ill may have greater difficulty recovering if they don't get enough sleep. It's ironic that hospitalized patients are awakened so frequently during the night (as illustrated by the standard quip "Wake up; it's time for your sleeping pill"). The people who might benefit most from uninterrupted rest are the very ones who are deprived of it and thus shortchanged on their recommended daily allowance of immunity.

With so little evidence that sleep has any significant and direct impact on tissues, organs, and processes outside the brain, we are back at square one—or rather, Theory #1: the notion that sleep, in large measure if not exclusively, is intended to revive and restore our cerebral function. For now, however, the real secret of why we sleep remains locked within the brain.

THE EVOLUTIONARY BASIS OF SLEEP

As a psychiatrist I have been exposed to many extreme forms of human behavior. I know of people who have gone without food for weeks at a time, whether compelled to do so in support of a moral cause or as the victim of mental illness. Some have reached the brink of starvation; others have fallen over it. I know, too, of homeless people who manage to survive for years without shelter. And there are many who forswear sexual activity for their entire lifetime, in answer to a religious calling or out of some deep-seated, pathological abhorrence. Food, shelter, sex: seemingly basic, vital needs which some people somehow manage to suppress for varying periods of time for one reason or another.

I know of no one, however, who has sworn off sleep forever— and made good on the promise.

Clearly we humans, like all other species of animals, have evolved a vital drive that compels us to sleep. And, as with most medical mysteries, researchers examine the animal kingdom for clues to our own behavior.

While it is known that all mammals sleep, their sleep patterns, like ours, are a reflection of their lifestyles and their environments. Imagine, for example, that you are a giraffe. If you knew it would take you ten seconds just to stand up and begin to run from an attacking lion, you would be pretty careful in choosing how and when you sleep. During the night a giraffe will experience full sleep—that is, lying on the ground, eyes closed, head rotated and resting on its thigh—only for brief periods ranging from a few minutes to an hour. The rest of the night is spent lying down but awake, or standing relaxed but alert. The giraffe's total time asleep is no more than about two hours a night, which seems to be an obligatory minimum; such a vulnerable animal does not have the luxury of indulging in optional sleep.

As evidenced by the giraffe, the need for sleep is not directly related to the size of an animal's body or the sophistication of its brain. Elephants, for example, sleep very little, while the small creatures of the night, like the bat and the opossum, may sleep more than ten hours a day. Herd animals—cows, sheep, horses— sleep in brief snatches; were they to sleep longer, they might awaken to find themselves separated from the herd and thus vulnerable to attack from wolves or other predators. Gorillas, who are hunted only by humans, sleep securely for more than sixteen hours a day. Sharks sleep very little; even while resting they must keep moving in order to keep oxygen-bearing water flowing through their gills. And since the blind Indus dolphin has to swim almost continuously in order to avoid injury in the turbulent waters that are its habitat, it is forced to limit its sleep to brief naps of less than ninety seconds, taken many times a day.

Another species, the bottlenose dolphin, gives new meaning to the phrase "half asleep," since one of the cerebral hemispheres of its brain sleeps while the other remains awake. After about an hour the two halves reverse roles. EEG tracings reveal that for the sleeping half the sleep is deep, with no signs of the rapid-eye-movement stage which signals the presence of dreaming. When the dolphin is fully conscious, both sides of the brain operate in full synchronization.

If we humans had somehow evolved this ability—to let one side of our brain doze off while the other remained active—the possibilities would be enormous. While the right side of the brain, responsible for abstract, creative expression, was dozing, we could use the left side, responsible for logical thought, to balance our checkbooks or write letters for an hour or so. Then the hemispheres could reverse roles; the right side could become activated, and we could devote our energies to painting or writing poetry while the left side caught up on its rest. The actual amount of our total "down time" could be limited to a few hours a night. Think of the progress the human species could make were it to add four more productive hours to its day!

Scientists generally assume that traits evolved by animals possess some kind of value in the struggle for survival. In other words, such traits—for example, the giraffes' long necks which enable them to eat the abundant leaves from the higher branches, or the bee's ability to perceive infrared light waves and thus detect hidden patterns on nectar-laden flowers—must contribute directly to the viability of the species. Otherwise they would have been jettisoned generations earlier as a waste of physiological resources. If this is true, the researchers argue, sleep must serve some essential role (although, as we have seen, exactly what the role is has yet to be established). Otherwise, why would a creature such as the bottlenose dolphin go to all the evolutionary trouble of devising such a complex sleeping arrangement?

Until more research is done, much of our thinking about sleep and its function will remain largely speculative. Sleep scientists pursuing answers are hampered by the fact no animal species has an EEG pattern equivalent to that of humans.

THE MECHANISMS OF SLEEP

Why we sleep is a difficult question to answer; *how* we sleep is not much easier. What happens when we fall asleep? Is it an electrical process, a shutting off of the circuits? Is it a chemical process, in which sleep-inducing chemicals are released by our brains to circulate and operate, like a team of secret agents? Is it a metabolic process, a form of collective bargaining by the organs of our bodies which demand a certain amount of time off from their life-giving labors? Again, the answers are unclear.

While modern researchers have not yet been able to identify

precisely the body systems that regulate sleep, their inquiries in recent years have focused on specific neural systems and chemicals within our brains. Interestingly, it appears that sleep is not one but two separate processes, each governed by different factors, which must occur simultaneously in order for us to fall asleep.

The Dewaking Process

This process involves the gradual shutting down of the systems that keep us awake or, in clinical terms, aroused. In preparing for sleep, our bodies begin turning down the receiving systems in our eyes, ears, and other organs, thus reducing sensory input to a minimum—just as we shut off the TV, turn off the lights, and calm things down so that our external environment will permit sleep to occur. Current theory holds that dewaking may be triggered by certain body chemicals, especially one known as GABA (gamma-aminobutyric acid), which apparently serve to reduce activity in certain parts of the brain. Much more research is needed to explain this process fully.

But just as a dark, quiet room is not in itself sufficient to put us to sleep, the reduced stimulation of our bodies is not adequate in itself to produce unconsciousness. Another process is needed to actually "manufacture" and distribute sleep to the now-receptive body.

The Sleep-Induction Process

This process involves changes in our body chemistry (specifically, brain chemistry) which serve to release the substances that actually put us to sleep. Scientists make a distinction between the factors that merely *facilitate* sleep, such as a good sleeping environment, sedative drugs, or a heavy meal, and the internal factors that *induce* sleep. These internal sleep-inducing factors are described as endogenous, which means they are built into our bodies and are not within our conscious control. The endogenous sleep-inducing factors are brain chemicals known as neurotransmitters. Once released, these chemicals circulate in our brains until they make contact with structures called neuroreceptors. Like a key fitting into an ignition switch, a neurotransmitter triggers (or "mediates") other activities, such as the release of more chemicals or activity by nerves.

The neurotransmitters associated with sleep are serotonin, norepinephrine, and dopamine. Of these the one that has been most thoroughly researched is serotonin. Sleep scientists theorize that serotonin plays the major role in inducing you to fall asleep after you have gone to bed. Once asleep, you progress through a cycle of various stages of deepening sleep, culminating in the rapid-eye-movement (REM) phase associated with vivid dreaming. As we'll see in the next chapter, each of these cycles may last about ninety minutes; you experience four or five cycles in a typical night's sleep. Serotonin is thought to be important in helping you to maintain sleep throughout the night, especially during the first thirty to sixty minutes of each sleep cycle, before you enter the REM phase. Besides being a sleep inducer in itself, serotonin may also act as a hormone—a chemical that alerts another organ, in this case the brain, to manufacture or release still other kinds of sleep inducers. In a sense serotonin may be compared to a military commander who can choose to fire the guns himself or order his troops to do the firing.

Another particular focus of interest is the hormone called melatonin. Produced by the pineal gland, located deep within the center of the brain, melatonin is a by-product that results when serotonin is acted on by other brain chemicals. Its production may also be the result of signals issued by the neurotransmitter norepinephrine. Experiments show that sleepiness is the most consistent principal effect of melatonin taken orally. It is thought that melatonin affects the same parts of the brain that react to drugs called benzodiazepines. These drugs—known as hypnotics, after Hypnos, the Greek god of sleep—are used in prescription sleeping pills and sedatives; I'll have much more to say about them in later chapters.

Interestingly, production of melatonin takes place largely in the absence of light. Consequently more melatonin is produced while we sleep at night. Levels of the chemical normally reach their peak just after midnight and fall to their lowest levels shortly after dinnertime. Thus, during those times of year when there are fewer hours of sunlight, more melatonin is produced; the more melatonin present in our bodies, the more we are likely to feel fatigued, unenergetic, and sleepy. One fascinating ramification of this research is the suggestion that increased melatonin production plays a role in causing the most common form of Seasonal Affective Disorder—the tendency to become depressed during the winter months.

Melatonin level in the blood or urine may also prove to be a useful indicator of other kinds of depressive disorders. We've seen that the onset of sleep requires both the reduction of arousal and the increase of sleep-inducing factors such as serotonin. It also appears that our progress through each ninety-minute cycle of sleep may itself be a similarly complex process, likewise triggered by changes in our brain chemistry. For example, some scientists suggest that one combination of brain chemicals is needed in order to start the REM period, while a second combination must be generated in order to bring REM sleep to a close. As with many other aspects of sleep, research in this field is not complete.

The roles played by neurotransmitters such as norepinephrine and dopamine are also subjects of controversy, due to the conflicting results of research on them. Nor is it certain what role other chemicals, such as the brain peptides, may play in the regulation of sleep. Further investigation in the coming years may reveal other fascinating aspects of the complex chemical stew that governs our every moment, waking or sleeping.

SLEEP DEPRIVATION: WHAT HAPPENS WHEN WE DON'T SLEEP

One method researchers have used to understand sleep is to study what happens to our bodies and minds when we are deprived of it. Although relatively few studies have been conducted, researchers have found surprisingly few negative effects of sleep deprivation in human experiments ranging in duration from three to eleven days. These effects are mostly minor and transitory and appear to pose no real long-term threat to health and well-being. For example, some people after two or three nights without sleep may experience hallucinations involving the senses of sight, touch, and hearing. Others may exhibit symptoms of paranoia or persecution, or a declining ability to function. These problems disappear, however, following a good night's rest.

Only minor physical changes have been reported as arising from acute, or short-term, lack of sleep. For example, there is basically no change in the physical ability to do work: you are still capable of lifting a normal load, although you may be unwilling to cooperate in doing so. Researchers have wondered whether the adrenal glands, which secrete certain hormones in response to stress, would demonstrate some kind of emergency response to a lack of sleep. So far, however, there is little evidence that they do so. I should note that total sleep deprivation has been known to kill laboratory rats, but only after a period of weeks.

One genuine risk of sleep deprivation is disruption of the circadian rhythms which control many of our basic bodily functions, a subject I'll return to in the next chapter. For example, even one night without sleep can throw off the timing mechanism that governs the release of stomach acid. Our bodies, awake at an odd hour, lose track of time and are fooled into believing that a meal is forthcoming; thus they begin the process of digestion even in the absence of food, resulting in the queasy, unpleasant sensation known as sour stomach.

With these few exceptions, then, it appears that no permanent physical side effects occur as a result of a few nights without sleep. Poor results on performance tests derive more from lack of willingness or motivation, or lack of challenging complexity in the required tasks, than from any physical decay. After three nights, incoherent speech, disorientation, and irritability do increase, but serious mental disturbances appear to be uncommon and, at worst, temporary.

For many years, in the absence of controlled studies, sleep researchers had to rely on anecdotal evidence about the effects of sleep deprivation. As a source for such evidence researchers in the early 1930s turned to the bizarre and sorry spectacle of the dance marathons.

Under marathon rules the hapless participants were limited in the amount of sleep time they could take: in the early days of a contest they were given a generous twenty minutes per hour. As the marathon wore on, however, the rules were changed to make the event more grueling by reducing sleep to ten, then five, then zero minutes in the final hours. Referees would disqualify contestants whose eyelids drooped for more than fifteen seconds, or who failed to take the required ten-inch steps.

After a few days of virtually nonstop staggering across the floor, some dancers began to experience hallucinations related to their extreme drowsiness. Others began to express strong paranoid feelings of persecution, suspicion, or mistrustfulness. In time the contestants would doze while dancing, depending on their partners to keep them upright and moving. Eventually, however, they would succumb to sleep and collapse on the floor, losing their chance at the prize money. (Incidentally, the record for participation in a dance marathon is held by a couple who lasted 214 days at a Chicago ballroom in 1930–31!)

A more scientific study of sleep deprivation took place in June 1933, when a man, known today only as "Z," decided that sleep was a waste of time and that he would break himself of the annoying habit. Two scientists were recruited to monitor his progress. By the third day Z began to report hallucinations; by the fourth he could no longer take a simple typing test due to his inability to focus on the page. Increasingly disoriented and argumentative, he became convinced he was being persecuted; by the tenth day he was unable to report any thoughts at all, and the experiment was terminated after 231 hours.

In 1959, as a fund-raising stunt, a radio disc jockey named Peter Tripp stayed awake for 200 hours. He seemed normal until the final days, when he began to experience auditory hallucinations and grew so paranoid that he refused to undergo any tests of his performance capabilities. (A few years later "The Dick Van Dyke Show" featured an episode based on the Tripp experience, in which Van Dyke slowly and comically dissolved into a blithering, bumbling wreck.)

A different experience was reported in 1964, when a seventeen-year-old California boy decided to set a record for sleep deprivation as part of his high school science fair. He managed to remain awake for eleven days without developing bizarre behavior patterns. The first night after the experiment was over he slept for fifteen hours, only eight more than usual. Within three days his sleep pattern returned to normal; he apparently suffered no permanent psychological or physical damage as a result of his ordeal.

So far you've been told that scientists aren't sure why we sleep or what exactly is the process that makes us sleep. At this point you might reasonably ask, "Well, what exactly constitutes 'normal' sleep?" My honest, if somewhat unsatisfying, reply is "It depends."

"NORMAL" SLEEP

How much sleep should you get each night? Without giving the matter too much thought, most people would answer eight hours. In fact, you may be reading this book because you find yourself sleeping for only five or six hours a night. At the other end of the scale, you may be lying in bed for ten or more hours a night and still feeling unrested.

There is no single answer about the amount of sleep a person needs. In my professional capacity I've met people, patients and colleagues alike, who thrive on five or six hours a night and others who need nine or ten. One co-worker of mine, a nine-hours-a-night man, knew full well what was disturbing his sleep: it was his wife, a television news writer, whose habit it was to awaken at four in the morning after only five hours of sleep. A novelist at heart, and not one to let those early hours go to waste, she would pound away furiously on her typewriter, turning out one gothic romance after another. Yet she functioned perfectly well throughout her busy, stressful day at work. My suggestion to the husband, which was unsolicited but which I'm told helped considerably, was to move her office into the farthest reaches of the house, soundproof the room, and wear earplugs.

These two people represent opposite ends of the sleep spectrum and make the point that, like so many other matters concerning personal health, sleep is the product of a number of variables. Someone who sleeps only five hours a night but is able to function happily during the day, feels rested, and does not suffer from unusual or troublesome medical conditions is obviously getting enough sleep. In contrast, another person may find that those same five hours of sleep represent a night of tossing and turning, leading to a day filled with fatigue and a decreasing ability to function on the job. Conversely, one ten-hour sleeper may sail through life perfectly well adjusted, while another finds that even that much time spent in bed provides too little rest and, to complicate matters even further, interferes with his family, social, and work life.

The Personalities of Sleep

There is some evidence that suggests a correlation between personality types and their sleeping patterns. Naturally your personality will have an impact on every facet of your life, sleeping as well as waking. If you tend to worry about every detail or event of the day, for example, you may indeed have trouble falling asleep. But the person who seems more relaxed and who takes things as they come without fretting unduly may also experience one form of insomnia or another, usually for some underlying medical reason.

Studies have found that some "Type A" people—those hard-driven, hyperreactive individuals—generally sleep for shorter periods of time each night than their more relaxed, laid-back "Type B" counterparts. Also, some people are known to cope with an increased level of stress in their lives by increasing the amount of time they spend asleep. Interestingly, these so-called "variable sleepers" have been found to exhibit the least amount of Type A behavior; thus their sleep patterns may be a crucial part of their mechanisms for coping with stress, which gives support to the notion that sleep helps recharge our batteries.

Another study has suggested that people who sleep less than the average tend to be more outgoing and friendly and may possess somewhat more conventional moral values. Conversely, the report adds, longer sleepers are often more introverted and demonstrate more individualistic and unconventional personalities; they may also tend to be more neurotic and to possess more of the traits associated with clinical depression.

As we will see throughout this book, however, sleep is affected by many different factors, including age, lifestyle, and personal habits. To ascribe a sleep disorder to an arbitrarily defined personality type can be misleading or, even worse, counterproductive when it comes to seeking an effective solution to the problem.

Are You Getting Enough Sleep?

In my practice I try to be sensitive to the true nature of a patient's complaint. For example, I often meet with patients once or twice a week for an hour, continuing these sessions over an extended period of time. During our conversations I usually hear frequent complaints about sleep: "I haven't slept a wink for days." "I tossed and turned all night." But if the patient appears to be well rested and wide awake, I know that we may be addressing the wrong issue. These patients are getting enough sleep, but for some reason they perceive themselves as insomniacs. Getting at the root of their problem takes time and persistence.

I generally measure the amount of sleep a person needs in terms of daytime alertness. My formula is simple: *If you go through the day wide awake, alert, and energetic, then you are getting enough sleep. If you do not, you may have a sleeping problem on your hands.*

Some scholars believe that the ancient Romans, with their passion for order and organization, created the notion that eight hours of sleep is the norm. It appears that, just as all Gaul was divided into three parts, so too were the Roman days, with one part devoted to sleeping.

Actually, the normal range for humans is between five and ten hours; the average worldwide is seven and a half per night. Only one person in a hundred can manage with five hours; another 1 percent needs ten. The rest of us mortals fall somewhere in between. (Of course, there are always exceptions. There are reports that a man in Spain was able to survive on less than an hour a day, while an English woman survived on just one or two hours. The verified record for short sleep, however, belongs to an Australian man who, despite only three hours of sleep per night, was able to function comfortably and efficiently during the day.)

Although no one is quite sure why, the amount of sleep you need, and the time you spend in bed, will be affected by where you live, how you earn your living, even the culture of your society. For example, a Gallup poll revealed that people in the eastern and midwestern states sleep less than those in the southern and western portions of the country. One explanation for such a difference may simply be the amount of time people in different areas need to commute to work. Obviously, if you face a two-hour train ride every morning, you're going to rise a little earlier than your counterpart in a small southern town, whose office is located a few miles up the road. The nature of your job can make a difference as well: a survey of Fortune 500 companies noted that almost 50 percent of the executives questioned reported that they sleep about six and a half hours a night. A third sleep more than seven hours, while 2 percent sleep between four and five hours. Such statistics, however, do not address a basic question: whether short sleep is a result of work pressures, or whether people who sleep shorter hours are naturally more likely to assume such high-pressure, high-profile positions.

Sleep Less—Live Longer?

Interestingly, long hours of sleep (nine to ten hours) do not necessarily lead to health and longevity. A study conducted by the American Cancer Society found that 99 percent of the adults who slept a "normal" average of seven to nine hours a night were still alive at follow-up six years later. The death rate of those who slept more than ten hours a night was nearly twice as high. The study also found that men who slept less than four hours had a mortality rate almost three times that of the "normal" group. This is not to say that sleeping too much or too little is in itself a threat to health; our bodies' mechanisms are far too complicated to permit such a simple conclusion. It is safer to interpret such statistics as indicating that physical and mental health problems can result in a number of symptoms, one of which is a poor sleeping pattern; left untreated, these problems can increase the risk of illness and death. It's also pertinent to note that, according to the study, the death rate among the group who used sleeping pills regularly was one and a half times higher than that of nonusers. Again, though, such statistics do not reveal whether the increased death rate arises from the pills themselves or from the underlying medical condition that may have led the person to use pills in the first place.

Several factors will affect the actual number of hours you sleep each night; perhaps the most important factor is your age. EEG patterns—the tracings of the electrical activity in your brain which can be interpreted to indicate the presence of sleep—are detectable in a human fetus long before birth. Some infants sleep over twenty-one hours on the first day after birth; some sleep only eleven hours. The average for a baby is about sixteen hours a day. By the time children are two or three years old, their total daily sleep averages about twelve hours. By the age of five, with school and other activities consuming much of the day, the daily nap is eliminated and the child needs about eleven hours of sleep.

As we age, a variety of factors affects the duration of our sleep. As children, between the ages of eight and seventeen, we are subject to increasing pressure, both academically and socially. What's more, the rigors of adolescence—rampaging hormones, maturing of the body, a range of new and conflicting emotions— can have a pronounced effect on sleep patterns. Strangely perhaps, children of this age group are now sleeping about an hour and a half less than their great-grandparents did seventy-five years ago. At least part of this change is attributable to social and scientific developments, such as the invention of the light bulb, and other factors including the increasingly early onset of puberty and the generally accelerating pace of living in the late twentieth century.

Beginning in our late teens, most of us average seven and a half hours of sleep per night. But at about the age of fifty we begin to sleep an hour less. Into the sixth decade and beyond, the effects of aging start to take a more serious toll: the organs function less efficiently. The cycles and systems that rule our sleep-wake patterns begin to deteriorate. It is a myth—common, but erroneous—that "old people need less sleep." More accurately, the elderly need the same amount of sleep as they did in their middle years, but their ability to sleep declines. An estimated 90 percent of Americans between the ages of sixty and eighty complain of chronic or occasional sleeplessness.

In studying EEG tracings, researchers have found that each of these changes in our sleep patterns as we age is associated with specific alterations in our nightly sleep cycle. For instance, among the elderly, that part of sleep that is deep, restorative, and without dreams almost completely disappears. A closer look at the cycle of sleep appears in the next chapter.

Besides age, your gender can make a difference in how you sleep, and for how long. More women than men get eight hours of sleep a night, but older women have a higher incidence of sleep problems than older men. Some sleep disturbance can be attributed to changes in hormonal balance which occur during the menstrual period, during pregnancy, and after menopause.

"Normal" sleep is not simply one long uninterrupted snooze. In a typical night you may shift position forty to seventy times. And if another person is sleeping with you in the same bed, the chances are that if you move, so will the other person, usually within twenty seconds. Such constant shifting is not a sign of disturbed sleep. On the contrary, it provides real benefit, as it prevents pooling of blood in your inert body, keeps the exchange of blood gases constant, and helps maintain muscle tone.

In a seven-hour period, the typical twenty-five-year-old will awaken only ten times. In contrast, if you are a senior citizen—more sensitive to the effects of snoring, noise, or involuntary movements—you may awaken over 150 times a night. Not all of these arousals result in attaining consciousness. More than likely you will stir, perhaps even open your eyes, but will return to sleep, none the worse for wear. Researchers believe that you must be awake for about ten to fifteen seconds before you become actually aware of what's going on around you. If you experience too many of these microarousals, however, you may find yourself feeling excessively sleepy on the following day. Such sleepiness can be a sign that something is wrong with your sleep, as we'll see in subsequent chapters.

Children who sleep for about nine and half hours are actually asleep for about 95 percent of their time in bed. As you probably know if you have ever tried to rouse a sleeping child, most youngsters seem to be able to sleep through almost anything. Perhaps such deep, uninterruptable sleep is a defense mechanism created by the immature central nervous system to protect its process of development. However, the percentage of time spent awake during the night, like the total amount of time we spend asleep, changes as we age. One study, for example, examined three groups of men of different ages. Those in their twenties, who slept for about seven hours, awakened an average of three and a half times per night and were awake about 1 percent of the time. By contrast, those in their forties slept six and a half hours, awakened nearly five times, and were awake about 6 percent of the night. The group in their seventies slept an average of six and three-quarters hours, awakened over seven times per night, and lay awake roughly 16 percent of the time.

As we can see, a "normal" night's sleep depends heavily on whether you are, for example, a "normal" twenty-five-year-old man or a "normal" seventy-year-old woman. In addition, the amount of sleep you need is determined primarily by your ability to function during the day.

Obviously, the gauge of your ability to function during the day is highly subjective. However, the following questions may help you assess your situation. In considering these questions, you should refer to your replies to the self-assessment section (pages 16–23).

* Has your boss complained about the quality or productivity of your work?
* Have you increased your coffee consumption, or do you find yourself needing coffee or other stimulants to get through the day?
* Do you feel more tired and less energetic now than you used to feel?
* Have family or friends complained about your lack of energy?
* Has there been a change recently in the number of hours you sleep each night?

If you answer yes to any of these questions, you may not be getting the "normal" amount of sleep for you.

In the next chapter we'll look at the complex rhythms and cycles that govern our sleep, and discuss ways in which you can evaluate your own sleep patterns.

4

Sleep Patterns

At some point in my medical education an instructor showed a film of a sleeping man. The time-lapse film, shot from the point of view of a fly on the ceiling, condensed eight hours of sleep into about three minutes and by doing so made it appear that the man hardly slept at all. He thrashed around in a seemingly continuous effort to find a comfortable position, now on his back, now on his side. He threw his covers off and pulled them back up again. He twitched; he kicked. The effect was almost comical. The point the instructor made, however, was an important one: Despite nearly constant activity the man in the film had experienced a typical, healthy, refreshing night's sleep.

As I have noted, sleep is not a single, uninterrupted event that begins when we shut our eyes and ends when we awaken in the morning. On the contrary: over the course of the night, we pass through a series of discrete sleep stages, each of which generates its own unique pattern of brain activity and changes in body function, and each of which serves a different function within the sleep process.

You may have noticed that you have a surprisingly consistent tendency to wake up every ninety minutes or so, but that on most occasions you are able to fall back to sleep. Or you may be aware that the dreams you have in the hour or two before you rise are longer, more complex, and more likely to be remembered than the ones you had earlier in the night. These sleep patterns are normal and reflect the wondrously complex structure (many experts use the apt term "architecture") of a night's worth of sleep.

Researchers have identified five distinct *stages* of sleep. Together these five stages make up one sleep *cycle*, which takes about an hour and a half to complete. Once we have passed through all of the stages, we experience a brief period of arousal, then begin the cycle over again. In a normal night of sleep, we will experience four or five of these cycles. What's particularly intriguing, as we'll discover shortly, is that each cycle contains a slightly different mix of the five sleep stages. Early in the night, for example, we will experience only a few minutes of dream sleep; later we may dream for an hour or more.

These sleep cycles, like many other physiological functions, appear to be governed by a kind of internal clock that regulates such processes as the release of hormones and fluctuations in body temperature. In recent years the discovery of this important regulating mechanism has led to the creation of a new branch of science called chronobiology, which examines the effects of time on organic systems.

In this chapter we'll take a closer look at the various stages of sleep and discuss the role our internal clock plays in helping us to maintain our state of health. Understanding the ways these intricate, complex mechanisms operate (and sometimes break down) can help lead to an understanding of why sleep problems arise—and how to correct them when they do.

STAGES OF THE SLEEP CYCLE

In the 1920s investigators using electroencephalogy found that the brain's electrical currents changed when the senses were stimulated. They also noted that epileptic seizures produced abnormal brain activity. Such results provided early clues that the study of brain waves could help unlock the secrets of what goes on within our skulls and provide important information about the disruption of normal brain activity during illness.

In the early 1930s scientists began to examine brain wave patterns during sleep and discovered not only that the patterns were different compared to those of the waking state but that they changed and evolved as the night wore on. By 1937 scientists had identified four completely separate stages of sleep (which they numbered 1 through 4) plus a presleep stage, or Stage 0. In the early 1950s the rapid-eye-movement stage was discovered. So important is the REM stage that all other stages are grouped together and known collectively as NREM (or non-REM) sleep.

After we fall asleep, then, one complete cycle is made up of the four NREM stages plus a REM stage, in the following sequence:

$$1-2-3-4-3-2-REM$$

Generally an average young adult will pass through a complete cycle in seventy to one hundred minutes, repeating the pattern between four and six times each night. As we will see, however, the time spent in each stage changes over the course the night. And, as previously noted, our sleep patterns continue to change and evolve as we age; in the elderly, for example, there is little or no deep sleep.

Today research continues to illuminate and refine our understanding of these basic stages. Briefly, the stages of sleep, as determined by EEG readings, are defined as follows.

STAGE 0

This is the usually pleasant time of transition from wakefulness to sleep. During this period you lie inactive, with eyes closed, waiting for sleep to befall you. At this point the potential of your muscles to perform work (their "tone") is still high; there may be some involuntary eye movement. Meanwhile, your brain continues to produce steady low-amplitude alpha waves, typical of an alert but relaxed (or meditative) waking state.

The transition from this stage to Stage 1 may take anywhere

from a few minutes to a half-hour or more; thus, if you turn in at 11:00 you should be asleep by 11:10 or 11:30 at the latest. Much longer than that, and you may be considered to have a form of insomnia.

STAGE 1

At this point you have truly begun to sleep, although it is still considered to be light sleep. This stage lasts anywhere from about thirty seconds to seven minutes. Thus if you fall asleep at 11:30, you may complete Stage 1 at about 11:35. During this stage your eyes may move slowly and your muscles may continue to carry electrical signals. Your pulse and respiration become more even. Stage 1 accounts for between 5 and 10 percent of your entire night's sleep.

STAGE 2

This stage lasts about an hour. In our example you would complete your first trip through Stage 2 by about 12:30. During this stage you become totally unaware of your surroundings; if someone lifted your eyelids, you would not see. Your breathing, heart rate, body temperature, and metabolism diminish. Approximately half of your night is spent in Stage 2. Interestingly, less is known about this period than any other stage of sleep.

STAGES 3 AND 4

The onset of Stage 3 sleep is indicated by its primary EEG feature: high-amplitude delta (or slow) waves, accounting for 20 to 50 percent of wave activity. In Stage 4 the very large and jagged slow waves have complete dominance, occurring more than 50 percent of the time. This is deep, physically restorative sleep, and your physiological systems are at their most regular and lowest ebb.

Usually Stages 3 and 4 are grouped together and called slow-wave or deep sleep. These periods range in duration from a few minutes to an hour; they are longest during the first one to two hours of sleep and virtually disappear by the fifth hour, accounting for 10 to 20 percent of total sleep. You may thus experience about a half-hour of deep sleep at about 12:30, before passing on to the first REM cycle at about 1:00 A.M. Men begin to spend less time in the deep sleep of Stage 4 during their thirties, while Stage 4 time does not decrease in women until they reach their fifties. The amount of deep sleep can be enhanced by exercise but is usually decreased by psychoactive medications and alcohol.

Physiologically there is a general decrease in blood flow to your brain during NREM sleep. Other systems in your body change as well: the heart rate falls about 6 percent; blood pressure drops by about 10 percent. Your breathing rate and the amount of gas expelled from your lungs decrease. Your respiratory system also lessens in its response to mild increases in carbon dioxide in the blood. This is the period during which growth hormone is released.

It takes more effort to rouse you from sleep in Stage 4 than in any other stage. Interestingly, though, sleepwalking and other sleep disturbances such as bed-wetting and night terrors seem to be related to the deep sleep of Stage 4, especially during the first hour after onset of sleep. And when people are deprived of sleep, they will spend more time making up for lost Stage 4 sleep than any other phase, indicating that this stage may have more value in providing rest and restoration.

RAPID-EYE-MOVEMENT (REM) SLEEP

In the first cycle of the night you may spend ninety minutes or so in the first four stages, after which you enter the REM sleep stage, a period marked by dreams and physiological changes that can affect the quality of sleep.

As noted earlier, the length of time devoted to each stage changes as the night evolves and the cycles recur. For example, your initial REM episode begins about an hour after onset of sleep and lasts only about ten or fifteen minutes. In the wee hours of the morning, REM stretches to approximately an hour, with the NREM period shortened to accommodate the average ninety-minute cycle. Generally most of your nighttime awakenings occur at the end of REM episodes.

EEG tracings during REM sleep closely resemble those of consciousness. The primary characteristic of REM sleep, as reflected in its name, is the fact that your eyes dart about quickly beneath the lids, as though you were scanning a landscape filled with action and detail. At this point your muscles are largely unable to function though they may twitch spasmodically. Your blood pressure and heart rate change dramatically. Men experience erections, usually not related to the content of their dreams; women may also undergo some kinds of subtle genital stimulation, such as clitoral engorgement, but these signs are harder to detect.

Blood flow to your brain increases with the onset of the REM stage. Your heart rate stays about the same, but it may speed up or slow down depending on such factors as the content of your dreams. Your respiratory system also undergoes significant changes. During REM sleep your breathing becomes shallower, more rapid, and erratic. The loss of muscle tone also leads to partial collapse of the upper airway. What's more, the ability of your lungs to clear mucus by coughing or through other mechanisms is lessened, causing them to retain their secretions. This is one reason why many people suffer coughing fits on rising.

The physiological changes associated with sleep stages awaken some people but are for the most part unimportant in normal, healthy people. However, for those who suffer from such ailments as cardiovascular and respiratory disease, the ramifications are potentially life-threatening. As noted earlier, sleep-related cardiovascular changes may trigger stroke, heart attack, angina, cerebral hemorrhage, or irregular heartbeat patterns called arrhythmias. Patients with impaired respiratory function, such as those with asthma or chronic obstructive pulmonary disease, may also find their conditions worsening at night *and* worsening their insomnia. A major respiratory problem associated with sleep is the interrupted breathing called apnea, one of the major forms of insomnia, which I have already mentioned and will deal with in greater detail in the next two chapters.

REM Sleep: A Closer Look

The onset of REM sleep is a complicated process not yet fully understood, involving interaction among a number of structures and systems in the brain, including neurotransmitters, synthesis of proteins, and other mechanisms. There may even be two different processes, one that turns REM sleep on and another that turns it off, which must work together to create a complete REM stage; more research is needed to supply definite answers. It is known, however, that sufferers of fragmented sleep—a form of insomnia characterized by frequent wakenings—tend to be roused only during their REM periods.

When you enter the REM phase, your body may give a convulsive jerk or exhibit some other form of movement. As I've said, your heart rate, blood pressure, and respiratory function change and more closely resemble the waking state than they do any of the other NREM stages. The brain undergoes increases in temperature, blood flow, and oxygen consumption. The daily peaks of biochemical, physiological, and psychological activity also occur during this phase.

Interestingly enough, although electrical signals are being carried through your muscles, causing mild twitching, your body remains almost totally immobile. The muscles of your chin, for example, are slack and limp, more so than at any other point of the day. There is a decrease in tone especially in your laryngeal, head, and neck muscles. Researchers feel that without this benevolent form of sleep paralysis we might thrash about so much that we would awaken and lose the benefit of sleep. Freud theorized—and was later proved correct—that the absence of muscle activity helps prevent us from acting out our dreams. Such loss of tone, however, may contribute to problems of sleep apnea and snoring.

Erection of the penis is usually the first sign of REM onset in healthy men of all ages. These erections occur regardless of whether the sleeper has experienced orgasm prior to falling asleep and are not affected by any neurosis that may afflict the individual. Men in their twenties usually experience an average of four or more episodes of erection in the course of a night. The incidence declines with age, but even men in their seventies average two and a half episodes in a typical night.

One patient of mine, a retired radio announcer in his sixties, told me his wife had noticed his nocturnal erections and was angry that he seemed to experience (and enjoy) sexual dreams in which she apparently did not play a role. I helped resolve their conflict by explaining to her that this is a universal feature of REM sleep in men and is unrelated to the content of dreams. In fact, such involuntary sexual arousal is often assessed by doctors as a way of determining whether a patient suffers from true impotence—the physical inability to achieve and sustain erection—or whether there may instead be an emotional basis for the problem.

Although adults achieve REM sleep after a descent and rise through the other sleep stages, infants begin their sleep with the REM phase and spend about half of their total sleep time—in some cases eight or more hours a day—in REM sleep. On the other hand, REM occupies only about 20 to 25 percent of sleep, or a total of about two hours per night, in adults. REM periods grow longer as the night wears on; the final REM period may last about an hour and may thus account for half of the total REM sleep achieved on a given night.

Obviously, in a ninety-minute cycle, periods of deep sleep must adjust to accommodate the increasing REM stage, like subway riders scooting over to make room for a bulky passenger. About five hours into the night, therefore, as REM stages lengthen, we have pretty much achieved our daily allotment of deep sleep, together with about half of our REM sleep.

Why Do We Need REM Sleep?

Our bodies seem to insist that we get a certain amount of REM sleep, at least over the long term. Scientists have found that when we miss out on some REM sleep—when we must rise a few hours earlier to catch a plane or to comfort a crying child, for example—we make up for lost REM time, at least to some extent, on subsequent nights. This phenomenon, knows as "REM rebound," means that on the night following REM deprivation the amount of REM sleep may increase to 35 or 40 percent of total sleep time, tapering back to the normal 20 to 25 percent after two to five days have passed. On awakening, we may experience the disruption in our REM pattern as a general malaise or restlessness lasting for a few days, until our sleep cycle returns to normal. One conclusion drawn from the rebound phenomenon is that almost all of the time spent in deep sleep, and about half our REM time, is obligatory—that is, necessary for health. People deprived of REM sleep show changes in behavior or in mental state, including increased appetite, anxiety and irritability, and difficulty concentrating. The rest of our sleep seems to be optional.

REM sleep, and its accompanying dreams, may permit us to adapt to or deal with the day's threatening experiences, discharging the instinctual drives and responses that we've had to suppress during our waking hours. (I remember that a childhood friend told me that he used to dream that our draconian third-grade teacher was a baseball—and he was at bat!) Or it may be that REM sleep dreams allow our brains the chance to shuffle through the vast amounts of information we receive during the day, discarding the useless data, consolidating the rest, and sending it into the relatively permanent storage vaults of our memories. One controversial view holds that the effects of REM sleep make it easier for our brains to learn complex material, such as a foreign language. It has been found, for example, that if you are exposed to new information and subsequently allowed adequate REM sleep, you are more likely to retain that information the following day than if you were deprived of sleep. We'll learn more about the functions of dreams in Chapter 12.

Another school of thought holds that REM sleep stimulates the brain and is crucial in the development of the central nervous system, a theory that helps account for the rapid onset and long duration of REM sleep in newborns and infants. It has been found, for example, that a fetus in the final three months of development spends about half its time in REM sleep, while a newborn, as we have seen, experiences REM for about eight hours a day. REM sleep may also play an important role in protein synthesis in the cells and may be necessary in the process known as anabolism, during which simple substances are converted into more complex living compounds.

One of today's foremost sleep researchers is Francis Crick, co-winner of the 1962 Nobel Prize for genetics, who holds that "REM makes our brain more efficient." It removes unnecessary connections between brain cells, connections which were formed during early development or as part of unimportant memories. In the process these modifications may flash through our brains and appear to us as dreams—sort of a cerebral waste-management program. This may account for the sometimes outrageous associations that appear in our dreams, as bits of vivid mental debris are collected, jumbled together in random fashion, and tossed into the psychic junk pile. In Crick's words, "REM allows us to function with smaller brains than we'd otherwise need if they remain cluttered with everything we've ever seen, heard, or felt. If we didn't have this process, we'd have more fantasy and get similar ideas mixed up, especially in childhood." This theory, however, like many theories about sleep, is controversial and awaits further experimental scrutiny.

WHAT DISTURBS REM SLEEP?

Other factors besides the aging process can influence our REM sleep amount. Disturbed REM sleep appears as a feature of numerous disorders both mental and physical. Following are details of the most common elements that can disrupt REM sleep.

Alcohol

A disturbance in the REM pattern can result from alcohol consumption. To illustrate the problem, let me tell you about a patient of mine, a grocery store manager in his forties who was plagued with nightmares. In one of our early conversations he revealed that he consumed two or three drinks at bedtime. Without them, he said, his dreams would be even worse and he'd be too scared to get into bed at night. I pointed out to him—much to his disbelief—that it was very possible that the alcohol itself was contributing to, if not actually causing, the problem.

I explained that the presence of alcohol in the blood tends to prevent the body from reaching the REM stage of sleep, especially during the first two or three ninety-minute sleep cycles. After five hours or so, the alcohol has been absorbed and eliminated by the body, and REM sleep returns in a somewhat more intense form. As discussed earlier, REM can rebound and take up more than its usual allotment of time, which means it must steal from the time given to other stages of the cycle. The sleeper thus enters a longer and intensely concentrated REM stage complete with vivid dreams, often with negative or frightening content. What's more, the sleeper is deprived of adequate time in the other, more obligatory stages and thus loses out on proper rest.

In those extreme cases where drinking binges last for days, or when a drinker finally withdraws from alcohol, REM sleep may have been suppressed for so long that eventually it can no longer tolerate being ignored. It then rebounds with a vengeance. Some investigators feel that the "DTs"—delirium tremens, with its symptoms of trembling, anxiety, and hallucinations—may be some form of the REM cycle that forces its way into the brain even while the drinker is awake.

This patient's case was a complicated one—it turned out that there were more reasons for his drinking than merely to prevent bad dreams. But by understanding the impact that his nightcaps were having on his nightmares, he was better able to cut back on bedtime alcohol consumption. The improvement in his sleep pattern, plus the greater sense of restfulness during the day, made him more responsive to the other steps in his therapy.

Depression

Abnormal sleep cycles are also a feature of clinical depression. In depressed patients more time is spent in Stage 1 sleep, while the amount of deep sleep (Stages 3 and 4) is reduced. The first REM stage occurs much sooner and is longer and more active than in normal individuals, whose long REM period occurs much later in the night. Because of this accelerated and foreshortened sleep cycle, depressed people often wake in the small hours of the morning, having completed their REM periods just as other people are beginning their longest dreams.

Narcolepsy

Some victims of narcolepsy, a condition characterized by uncontrollable daytime sleep attacks, are unable to keep REM sleep "in its place." Their sleep usually omits the slow-wave periods and begins with a REM phase which, as we've seen, does not usually occur in healthy adults for an hour or more. The percentage of REM sleep in narcolepsy is normal, but the REM is fragmented, shattered into smaller units and appearing at different points in the day instead of in the normal pattern.

REM-Interruption Insomnia

Although we'll be discussing the various types of insomnia in subsequent chapters, it's worth mentioning at this point that there is a form of sleep disturbance specifically related to the REM period. In this disorder, known as REM-interruption insomnia, sleepers—usually men over thirty-five years old—are aroused during the first REM stage of the night, after the stage has been firmly established. They continue to awaken in at least three out of every four REM periods, again at a point well into the cycle. Frequently victims are unable to fall back asleep, thus losing as much as four to six hours of sleep a night. This form of insomnia is usually linked to an emotional disturbance caused by depression or traumatic events. The awakenings may be caused by a sudden flurry of eye movements, perhaps as the result of vivid or troubling dreams. It often happens that someone who has recently suffered a nightmare tends to awaken to avoid a repeat occurrence. Such disruptions in the REM cycle can aggravate other symptoms of mental disturbance, such as depression or paranoia.

CIRCADIAN RHYTHMS: THE BODY'S OWN TIME ZONE

Recently a patient of mine, an advertising account representative in her thirties, described herself as being "absolutely, positively incapable of functioning until noon on Monday." Unfortunately, her boss insisted on scheduling crucial management planning sessions at ten o'clock on Monday mornings. More so than most people, she found that time difficult, especially after an active weekend of socializing. She felt that her "Monday blues" had caused her to miss out on a much-desired promotion. I suggested that it was her weekend schedule that was affecting her job performance. Working together, we formulated a plan that involved a carefully regulated schedule of weekend bedtime (midnight or 1:00 A.M., depending on how sleepy she felt) and, more important, a strict rising time of 8:00 A.M. on Saturday and Sunday. Although such a schedule demanded compromises in her social life, she found that with the support of her sympathetic lover she was able to implement the plan and stick to it. Monday mornings are considerably less difficult, she reports, although she admits "it is still hard to smile at anyone until ten-thirty at the earliest."

Why did this adaptation work?

Most people possess a natural, twenty-five-hour circadian clock which they must constantly adjust to life based on the twenty-four-hour reality of the earth's rotation. Realistically this arrangement means we generally go to bed an hour earlier than our bodies would prefer. Come the weekend, however, we are usually freed from any imposed schedules and tend to go to bed an hour or so later on Friday night and perhaps two hours later on Saturday. On Sunday night, knowing we have to work in the morning, we return to a conventional cycle. We try to force ourselves to sleep at perhaps eleven o'clock when our bodies, spoiled by indulgence in the previous forty-eight hours, would rather turn in closer to two or three o'clock. Thus we drag ourselves out of bed Monday morning at seven, after perhaps eight hours in bed but about four hours earlier than our circadian "factory manager" would prefer. No wonder the "Monday morning blues" are such a common phenomenon!

In recent years the term "circadian rhythm" (those rhythms that govern our circadian clock) has been applied to a growing number of metabolic and other patterns found in virtually all creatures. These discoveries led to the creation of the new science of chronobiology.

The first experiments to discover and assess the circadian rhythms in humans were conducted in Europe in the early 1960s. German researchers used the basement of a Munich hospital to isolate volunteers from all external time clues (called *Zeitgeber*, a German neologism that means "time giver"). There were no windows, nor were the subjects permitted to see newspapers or hear radio or television broadcasts. The participants in the experiment were allowed to establish and follow their own schedules, eating when they were hungry, sleeping when they felt tired. In similar fashion French scientists a few years later used caves in the Alps to isolate their subjects. Among other things, these experiments showed that, left to their own devices, the volunteers tended to go to sleep at twenty-five-hour intervals.

This and subsequent discoveries have established that human circadian rhythms, when allowed to run free with no clues to establish the time of day, tend to operate on a cycle of approximately twenty-five hours. One ramification of this finding is that if our circadian pacemakers were not reset on a daily basis by external factors, the timing of our built-in rhythms would be off by an hour more each day compared with time as measured by the clock.

Circadian rhythmicity appears to be characteristic of virtually every physiological process and function, including body temperature, the secretion of hormones, sleep, hunger, mood, alertness, and sexual desire. For example, body temperature and the ability to perform efficiently on certain simple tasks dip to their lowest point in the early hours of the morning, as we sleep, and reach their maximum point in the evening. On the other hand, cell division and the secretion of certain hormones are highest during the night, while measurements of adrenaline and noradrenaline concentrations and such mental skills as concentration normally reach a maximum at about midday. So ubiquitous are these rhythms that body functions without demonstrated rhythmicity have proved to be the exception, not the rule.

Some rhythms even seem to anticipate periodic events, such as dawn or dusk. Body temperature, for example, begins to rise shortly before waking. Experiments have shown that if an animal is trained to expect a meal at a certain time every day, the enzymes in its gastrointestinal tract will begin to show activity in advance of actual feeding.

The time needed to complete one cycle of a given body rhythm—its period—can vary from a tiny fraction of a second to as long as a year or more. Circadian rhythms are those that require approximately a day to complete. (The word "circadian" is derived from the Latin *circa*, meaning "about," and *dies*, meaning "day." A year-long rhythm might technically be described as "circannual.") Most people recognize those biological rhythms with a high frequency, such as a heartbeat (about sixty to eighty times a minute). The longer ones are less obvious, since they need to be observed over a period of days or even years.

The Role of Circadian Rhythms

It is now believed that one major role of the circadian timing system is to organize our bodily processes and systems so that they occur in the proper sequence. In this way those functions that depend on each other can be coordinated, and those that are incompatible or that might interfere with each other can be separated. As suggested above, I like to think that the circadian system acts as a factory manager who schedules workers, arranges the delivery of goods, determines production, and orders shipment of final products so as to achieve maximum efficiency. To demonstrate the point, let's assume that a high body temperature is incompatible with secretion of a given hormone. The circadian pacemaker might coordinate the lowering of temperature so that, among other reasons, the hormone can be released to function properly. The pacemaker allows enough time for the hormone to complete its task, then brings the temperature back up to enable other body functions to operate at their peak. This is admittedly a simplified example, but it illustrates the point.

Jet lag, which was covered in greater detail earlier (pages 51–58), appears to be largely the result of disruptions in our circadian cycles caused by our attempts to adjust suddenly to a new time zone. There are other, potentially more serious ramifications as well. It has been shown, for example, that one- and two-car accidents tend to occur, not during rush hour as you might expect, but at those times of day (between midnight and 7:00 A.M. and between 1:00 and 4:00 P.M.) which coincide with certain low points in our physiological function. Some researchers attribute this statistic, at least in part, to those circadian rhythms which dominate during these hours and which tend to make us vulnerable to unwanted sleep. Also, investigators ascribe some airline crashes to the circadian disruptions that are a known occupational hazard for pilots on long flights or flights at odd hours. And in the previous chapter I mentioned the fact that some cardiac diseases and other afflictions such as cranial hemorrhage are more likely to strike during the night, while some of our circadian defenses are down.

At this point it might be well to note that circadian rhythms—a known and accepted physiological principle—are not the same as "biorhythms," a fad that reached its peak in the 1970s. While circadian rhythms dominate our every bodily function, biorhythms were declared by some to be long-term cycles of physical and emotional health that could be traced back to the date of birth and, at least theoretically, used to project our performance on any given day. "Computers" designed to generate biorhythm charts appeared in shopping malls, restaurants, movie theater lobbies, and turnpike rest stops. In exchange for a quarter the machines purportedly warned people that they would reach a peak or a trough on such and such a day, that they should avoid driving or sexual contact, and so on—sort of a high-tech form of palm reading. Not surprisingly, biorhythms were dismissed as pop science by chronobiologists. In one study, for example, investigators compared reports of thirteen thousand on-the-job accidents, as well as eighty-five hundred airplane mishaps, with the so-called critical days supposedly predicted by the biorhythms of the workers and pilots. No correlation was found.

There are a number of factors that can alter the circadian rhythms and disrupt the normal pattern of body functions. Illness is one major factor. Adjusting to daylight saving time is another: we arbitrarily begin operating on a longer or shorter day. It may take a few days for our systems to become entrained to the new cycle. Similarly, at the conclusion of a weekend, many people (like the advertising representative I described earlier) may say they are suffering from "Monday morning blues," known technically as acute circadian phase disruption. Their self-prescribed therapy is to ingest massive doses of caffeine in the form of coffee, in an attempt to jump-start their mental and physical motors. Aging also affects the internal clock as the organs begin failing to work in harmony. People who have retired or who have fewer social contacts may lack the social time cues to which they had grown accustomed.

Shift workers are particularly prone to phase disruption. One of my patients, a fifty-year-old dispatcher for a taxi company, preferred to work the midnight shift because it suited his wife,

a nurse who also worked at night. He found that every two or
three weeks or so he went through a period when he was virtually unable to stay awake on the job. I scoured medical literature
on the subject and was surprised to learn that people in his
situation frequently go through phases of extreme and disabling
sleepiness. One solution, discussed in greater detail in Chapter
2, involves rotating shifts on a weekly basis: working midnight
to 8:00 one week, then 8:00 A.M. to 4:00 P.M., then 4:00 to midnight. Although many workers dislike rotating shifts, preferring
to maintain a constant work pattern, my patient tried this approach successfully; there were some difficulties with his wife,
but she too was eventually able to adjust her schedule. It is more
often the case, however, that shift workers lack the power to
structure their own schedules, and other solutions must be
found.

Circadian Rhythms, Sleep Disturbance, and Illness

Our basic circadian cycle of sleeping and waking is built into
our systems as a product of our genetic inheritance. The actual
rhythm of the cycle is not established until sometime after birth,
when the central nervous system is more fully developed. This
sleep-wake cycle is the result of a number of processes that must
work together in close harmony.

With such intricate mechanisms involved, it is perhaps not
surprising that so many of us suffer from occasional inability to
sleep. In fact, an entire class of sleep disorders, known as disorders of the sleep-wake schedule, all involve misalignment between people's daily routines and their internal circadian
rhythm. Circadian disruption is a likely suspect in those cases
where a patient has an erratic sleep schedule or complains of
inability to fall asleep. Such people often describe themselves as
night owls.

Moreover, the sleep-wake cycle itself affects a number of processes, and some researchers believe that it may be connected to
the onset and intensity of disorders such as anxiety or depression. For example, studies have linked the abnormal EEG tracings of depressed people to disturbances in the biological

rhythms. These rhythms apparently occur earlier than normal in the cycles of depressed patients.

Circadian rhythms can have a profound impact on other chronic diseases. One of the most familiar examples, perhaps, is nocturnal asthma, also known as "nighttime wheeze." That the severity of asthma can worsen at night has been known for centuries. Nighttime attacks were attributed to a variety of causes, from too many bedclothes to feather bedding and bedbug bites, before more scientific research in recent years implicated circadian rhythms. For example, the dimensions of breathing pathways in the throat and lungs and the ability of air to move in those pathways are known to change at night, in normal people as well as in asthmatics. But in large measure these changes are rhythmic, following a definite circadian pattern that is actually the net result of the effects of other rhythms. For example, the levels of the circulating compounds that act to stimulate the heart, lungs, and other organs reach their lowest levels at night. At the same time, the sensitivity of the bronchial system to allergens is at a maximum. Immunological activity and clearance of mucus by the lungs also exhibit rhythmic patterns. Normally these various rhythms present no problem. For the asthmatic, however, the rhythms seem to conspire to make asthma worse at night. (Low levels of some of these same compounds and low immunological activity also play a role in increasing the severity of rheumatoid arthritis during the first few hours after waking.)

Clearly, those of us who can take a night of sleep for granted are very lucky. With the fine balance between NREM, REM and circadian rhythms, it's amazing that even more people don't suffer from sleep disorders. Similarly, the complexity of our sleep can make treating sleep disorders difficult. In the next chapter we'll look at the reasons why so many of us do have trouble falling or staying asleep.

5

Difficulty Falling or Staying Asleep

Insomnia takes many forms, each as different from another as—well, as night and day. In my years of clinical practice I've seen thousands of patients with sleep disorders, and no two of them have ever had exactly the same symptoms or responded to exactly the same therapeutic approach.

As new data from sleep research continue to pour in, the medical world must continually revise its concept of what constitutes a sleep disorder. Predictably, much confusion exists over definitions, terms, and classifications. Small wonder, then, that some physicians, inundated by the growing flood of information about all aspects of medicine, may have a difficult time keeping up with developments in this particular field and may thus be unaware of the newest techniques for identifying a particular sleep disturbance and the latest approach to designing an effective treatment strategy.

Many forms of insomnia combine elements of psychological, organic, and emotional disturbance, elements that are further exacerbated by styles of living, patterns of behavior, and environmental factors over which the patient may have little control. Thus a physician must assemble an array of information about your condition before correct assessment can be made. For example, questions about your sleeping patterns in childhood may shed a surprising amount of light on your current problem. In addition to sleep and family histories, your sleep diary will help to illustrate current nocturnal patterns. Other pertinent details will be gleaned from a history of drug use, prescription and otherwise. A medical history and physical exam not only will serve to establish whether an organic condition exists that may be contributing to your problem but will in most cases reassure you that your health is not currently suffering due to lack of sleep. A detailed psychiatric history is perhaps the single most important component of the patient profile. While confusion exists about many aspects of insomnia management, there is virtually unanimous agreement that the majority of insomnia cases—as many as 80 percent—have a psychological component that must be addressed if therapy is to be effective.

Even with complete medical and psychological information it is possible to misinterpret the findings. Reports indicate that a physician may miss clues suggesting a physiologic cause of insomnia in as many as three out of ten patients. What's more, the doctor who relies solely on the patient's description of the problem may overestimate the degree of sleeplessness in one or two out of ten cases. As we've seen, insomnia victims often remark that they "didn't sleep at all" when laboratory findings indicate otherwise.

Remember that insomnia is not so much a disorder as it is a symptom, one that stems from any number of causes. Nor is it merely a measurement of the number of hours of sleep experienced on a given night. The pattern of sleep disruption and the resulting quality of sleep are critical elements: when did sleep occur and when was it interrupted? Was it deep and restorative or light and fragmented? Armed with these facts, the physician can begin to penetrate the darkness.

Popular media, including television, magazines, and the tabloids, only add to the confusion about insomnia. Advertising often portrays a world in which sleep problems disappear after merely taking a pill. And articles aimed at the layman may oversimplify or misstate the nature of insomnia. One recent publication invented a set of clumsy names—as if more were needed—for the

various types of sleep disorders. For example, the inability to fall
asleep promptly was called "initardia." Other varieties were
given such names as "pleisomnia," sleep interrupted by awakenings; "scurzomnia," short sleep; "hyperlixia," excessive light
sleep; and "turbula," sleep laden with uneasy dreams.

Naturally, as a physician, I prefer to use the more precise, if
less colorful, terminology agreed upon by experts who, over the
last dozen years or more, have wrestled with the problem of
identifying and classifying sleep problems. Precise categorization is not simply an exercise in academics—far from it. The
symptoms of different forms of insomnia may appear to be very
similar on the surface; patients may even use the same phrases
in describing them to a physician. Their causes, however, may
be radically different. To cite a parallel example: you may sneeze
because of an allergy to dust, or because you are infected with
a cold virus. While the symptom sneezing is the same, the causes,
as well as the remedies, are completely different. By the same
token, therapies that work for one form of sleep problem often
prove to be ineffective—or worse, counterproductive—for another.

With that in mind, then, this chapter will be devoted to a
discussion of the first major category of insomnias: the disorders
of initiating and maintaining sleep, or DIMS.

Generally, DIMS includes those conditions responsible for
creating disturbed or insufficient sleep. These disorders are distinct from those that cause excessive daytime sleepiness or disrupt the normal circadian cycle of sleeping and waking. As we
will see, however, their symptoms and their effects on health and
performance may be much the same.

The DIMS category accounts for approximately 30 percent of
all cases of sleep disturbance. DIMS consists of four major
groups:

* Disorders caused by a conditioned response or negative expectations about sleep
* Disorders caused by medical, environmental, psychiatric, or
  alcohol or drug problems
* Disorders caused by breathing or muscular irregularities
* Disorders arising from true organic insomnia (a very rare
  condition)

DIMS takes many forms: difficulty falling asleep initially, frequent wakenings, trouble returning to sleep once aroused, waking too early in the morning. The pattern of the disturbance is crucial in diagnosis, because it can help to differentiate DIMS from other categories of disorder. For example, disturbances caused by patients' emotional or environmental situations tend to prevent them from crossing the threshold of sleep. In contrast, victims of endogenous depression are subject to awakenings that occur in the early hours of the morning.

FEATURES OF DIMS

Difficulty falling asleep—initially as well as after nocturnal awakenings—is the single most frequently reported complaint of insomniacs, regardless of age or sex. Sometimes lifestyle has much to do with this problem. Obviously, you can't eat a rich meal at ten o'clock at night, in a lively restaurant atmosphere in the company of boisterous, stimulating people, and expect to drop off easily at midnight. But there may be other, more subtle reasons for your problem. (The problem of "dropping off" is different from a disorder known as delayed sleep phase syndrome, a disruption of the circadian system that causes a person to feel sleepy hours later than normal; this condition will be covered in Chapter 6.)

Interrupted sleep usually appears after the age of forty. All of us wake several times during the night; usually these wakings do not stir us to the point of consciousness. In clinically significant cases, however, patients wake more and more frequently and for longer periods of time. Once aroused, they may begin to ruminate—"Now I'll never get back to sleep"—which only compounds the problem. Causes of these awakenings may range from fear of intruders (with subsequent sensitivity to every creak and rustle heard in the night) to chronic unexpressed anger. Depression may also be involved. One primary reason for awakenings in the elderly is their inactivity during the day, coupled with naps that tend to rob them of nocturnal sleepiness and with a general tendency to sleep lightly anyway. And, of course, the elderly are prone to chronic conditions such as arthritis, heart disease, or breathing abnormalities, any one of which may play a role. Frequently, too, they take a variety of medications which may wreak havoc on their sleep patterns.

Early-morning insomnia causes you to wake too soon, before sufficient sleep has been achieved, and is coupled with an inability to fall back asleep. As we've seen, truncated sleep can stem from depression or circadian disruption; it may be related to other disturbances in the sleep cycle, especially the REM phase. Earlier I discussed the role of alcohol in causing foreshortened sleep. Ironically, another reason for early waking may be the use of a benzodiazepine sleeping pill with a short duration of action, such as triazolam. When the effects wear off, wakefulness returns sooner than is desirable.

PROFILE OF A DIMS INSOMNIAC

The sleep-wake pattern is the first clue to a diagnosis of DIMS. In addition, the length of time a disorder has persisted—a few days? years?—is a significant factor in understanding the problem. All of us suffer disturbed sleep at some time or another as a normal response to grief, illness, or a major change in our lives. A long-term sleep disruption, however, may be the result of behavioral patterns learned in childhood. This kind of conditioned response accounts for perhaps a third of all DIMS diagnoses.

Like other physicians I have noticed other patterns of behavior common to many insomniacs. They frequently report that, come bedtime, they feel increasingly tense and anxious. They begin to ruminate about the state of their health, their problems at work, or their personal relationships. Thoughts of death intrude. I've already mentioned that common but bizarre prayer "Now I lay me down to sleep"; the scientific literature on sleep contains reports of people who have been terrorized by this innocent prayer and its not-too-concealed threat that they might die before they awaken. One sensitive parent I know of rewrote the prayer this way: "In the morning when I wake, keep me again for thy dear sake," thus effectively shielding her children from the association between sleep and death.

In large measure, insomniacs are people who lack adequate

means of dealing with stress, who tend to turn their emotions inward. Laboratory studies demonstrate that these thought patterns have physiological consequences in that they stimulate the autonomic nervous system. Heart rate, muscle tension, and body temperature may increase, making onset of sleep more difficult. In the morning these individuals feel worse than on retiring: tired, unrested, irritable. They drag themselves through the day feeling tense, unhappy, not fully in control.

I've also found that some insomniacs use their disorder as a mechanism to avoid certain issues or obligations in their personal lives. One of my patients, a thirty-six-year-old man I'll call Jim, had experienced difficulty falling asleep for nearly ten out of the twelve years he had been married. While his wife usually went to bed by 11:30, Jim would stay up for hours, finding a number of tasks, such as balancing the checkbook, that had to be done before he could turn in. He was convinced that he suffered from some kind of "chemical imbalance" that simply prevented him from enjoying normal sleep patterns; he believed that a prescription for sleeping pills was all he needed.

During one discussion, however, Jim made a casual remark to the effect that the birth control method he used was celibacy. To my surprise, I discovered that he had intercourse with his wife no more than half a dozen times a year. On further probing I learned that Jim suffered from deep-seated fears about his sexual performance, which apparently stemmed from some thoughtlessly facetious remarks his wife had made shortly after they were married. Eventually, it seems, his fears were transformed into a behavior pattern that kept him from going to bed at the same time as his wife, in order to avoid confronting the issue of sex and exposing himself to the risk of what he perceived as "further ridicule." After some encouragement and therapy Jim discussed these feelings with his wife, who, I am happy to say, cooperated by reassuring him about his sexual desirability and performance. At last report Jim's sleep pattern—as well as his sex life—has returned to nearly normal.

As you can see from this example, Jim subconsciously used his insomnia as a means of avoiding sexual confrontation. Similarly, other patients blame sleeplessness for poor performance at work or use it to minimize expectations people might have of them or to avoid risk of failure. Still others find they can avoid family or social obligations by using their chronic fatigue as a constant excuse.

In some cases, of course, DIMS stems not from psychological causes but from a true organic abnormality, such as a disruption in the nervous system responsible for controlling breathing. Complicating matters is the fact that such organic insomnia often mimics the symptoms of psychological insomnia, especially when the problem is one of interrupted sleep. Organic sleep disturbance seldom results in premature morning waking—an example of why a detailed understanding of an individual's sleep pattern is so important in diagnosis. To reiterate, however, a psychological element will be found in most cases of insomnia.

TYPES OF DIMS

Let's look now at the specific types of DIMS.

As I indicated earlier, the length of time a sleep disorder has persisted is an important element in understanding the nature of the problem and in prescribing treatment. Consequently, sleep problems in the DIMS category (and other categories, for that matter) are further classified as being transient (lasting only a few days), short-term (from one to three weeks), or long-term or persistent (a month or longer).

Transient DIMS is easily recognizable, even predictable, arising as it does from sudden or powerful—and, fortunately, relatively short-lived—emotional stress. The upheaval of such major life events as marriage, divorce, or the birth of a child can precipitate a sleep disturbance. Students facing exams are notorious victims. Other causes of transient DIMS include jet lag or hospitalization. As its name implies, transient DIMS lasts no more than a few days, perhaps a week.

Short-term DIMS lasts from one to three weeks and can also stem from emotional crisis, such as the loss of a job or a perceived threat from one source or another. Family stress, severe disappointments, frightening events, or illness often result in sleep disturbance that continues over the course of a few weeks. Diagnosis is relatively simple, in part because the patient usually reports a completely normal sleep history; however, people who are insecure and vulnerable to emotional arousal are at particular risk for this kind of sleep disorder. Also, short-term insomnias are likely to recur and often appear as a combination of patterns—for example, difficulty falling asleep plus early-morning awakenings—not usually seen in the more persistent forms.

As a physician, I sometimes breathe a silent sigh of relief when a patient comes to me with one of these complaints, since I know that the problem is likely to be temporary and will respond quickly and completely to any number of therapies. I don't want to downplay these forms of insomnia, because they are very real and very troubling for those who experience them. They are also very common, so much so that they are sometimes referred to as "insomnias of everyday life." In fact, left alone, the problem would in many cases simply resolve itself. However, the fact that a patient has turned to me for help means that I must take some action to alleviate the condition, even if it is only reassurance and support.

Sometimes simply talking about the situation provides great relief. If a loved one has died, for example, the patient may wish to be unburdened of thoughts of grief or hostility that cannot be expressed to friends or to other members of the family. In some instances I will prescribe low doses of a short-acting benzodiazepine hypnotic drug to induce sleep, usually asking the patient to take it for only a few days at a time. In Chapter 11, I describe the drugs available, their advantages and drawbacks; for now, let's say that while drugs can be helpful, I prefer to use them as sparingly as possible. One factor that affects my decision to use pharmacotherapy, especially in short-term DIMS, is whether I sense the patient is at risk of learning some kind of insomniac behavior, a pattern that may become reinforced over a relatively brief time. If so, I will intervene quickly to try to break the cycle before it becomes entrenched.

Persistent DIMS is a type of disorder that afflicts the patient for a month or more; as we've seen, this form of insomnia can last for years and is directly attributable to the learned behavior I've just described. For example, a patient may experience some kind of illness or emotional crisis that, among other symptoms, disrupts sleep. However, when the illness is cured, or after the crisis has passed, the insomnia may take on a life of its own and become the focus of the patient's concern. He or she then perceives the insomnia as a distinct disorder in itself.

The insomnia thus hangs on long after the initial, precipitating cause has disappeared; the longer the pattern continues, the more entrenched it becomes. Just entering the bedroom and experiencing its sights, smells, and sounds can trigger feelings of unpleasantness. Frequently the patient will conduct some kind of inner monologue: "Oh God, it's bedtime . . . another night of tossing and turning. I just know I'll never get to sleep. I hate this ritual. . . ." In this way victims reinforce their insomnia on a nightly basis, until it has swollen into a kind of sleep phobia. The technical term for this kind of conditioned disorder is "psychophysiological," a combination of syllables that appropriately suggests the impact the mind can have on the way the body behaves. According to one study psychophysiological factors are present in about half of all diagnoses of DIMS.

By carefully eliciting the patient's medical and psychological history, I find I can usually detect the conditioning pattern. Ruling out sleep disturbance stemming from medical conditions or psychiatric problems such as anxiety, fear, depression, or the form of neurosis known as obsessive-compulsive behavior, I begin to suspect that I am confronting a case of persistent DIMS. One key element in confirming the diagnosis is the patient's absorption with the sleep process itself, to the exclusion of other mental or emotional concerns. Often he or she reports desperate and self-defeating efforts to obtain sleep, revealing in the process the degree to which a sleep problem is overanticipated.

Some patients get themselves so worked up about sleep that they find it impossible to wind down at bedtime. I remember one who stayed awake at night reading every book and article he could find about sleep, trying to find the reason for his insomnia! This behavior also illustrates another symptom: as a rule, patients with persistent DIMS do not know (or perhaps they suppress knowledge of) the reasons for their inability to sleep. Compare this to patients with depression, who know all too well the basis of their early-morning insomnia.

Another clue to persistent DIMS is that its victims often find, to their surprise, that they are able to sleep better in a part of the house other than the bedroom. Similarly, they are much more likely to get a good night's rest as an overnight guest at a motel or the house of a friend—or even in a sleep laboratory. The reason for this is clear: by moving away from the room that triggers the negative associations and behaviors concerning sleep, the insomniac breaks the self-feeding cycle of sleep disturbance. Since there is no other basis for the insomnia—an organic abnormality, for example—the patient sleeps soundly.

In some cases insomnia is a desperate signal for help. Ironically, however, these patients may send out a simultaneous message that they cannot, or will not, be helped. When I suggest, for example, that something in their behavior may be contributing to the problem, a typical response may be "What, you think it's all in my head? It's not! I genuinely can't sleep!" Often when I propose that the patient undergo some form of psychological counseling, the reply is "Oh, that's no good. That won't work for me. I need a pill that will knock me out. That's the only thing that will do the trick."

If an insomnia is genuinely psychophysiological in origin, then no variety or quantity of drugs will do much good for long. Effective treatment involves counseling and therapy that supports and encourages the patient while attempting to break the pattern of reinforced behavior. I'll describe the options available in Chapter 10.

THE MANY FACES OF PERSISTENT DIMS

Psychiatric DIMS

There are other forms of persistent DIMS that are not products of bad habits. Depression accounts for the greatest incidence of chronic insomnia attributable to psychiatric disorders. It has been called the "common cold of mental health." Of course, a distinction must be drawn between clinical depression—a serious and sometimes debilitating condition—and sadness, which is a normal and transient reaction to unhappy experiences. The clinically depressed individual suffers a host of symptoms: anxiety, withdrawal from society, low energy, inability to function normally, loss of appetite and sexual drive. Often victims neglect their health and appearance. Physically they experience palpitations and shortness of breath. Their memory is poor, the ability to concentrate diminished; they are plagued with feelings of guilt, illogical thoughts, and a sense of isolation. Most patients with chronic insomnia show some type of depressed behavior; however, only a small percentage are actually diagnosed as having depression.

Not surprisingly, depression affects circadian patterns. Several rhythms, including body temperature and circulating cortisol, are abnormally advanced—they occur too soon—in the sleep-wake cycle. Secretion of prolactin and growth hormone is also affected. Some researchers feel that such disruptions in the various neuroendocrine rhythms could be related to the onset and intensity of mental illness. There may also be an association between the incidence of depression and the year-long cycle of melatonin. Statistics indicate that hospital admissions for depression are higher when patients have reached the low point in their annual melatonin rhythm.

As I've said, virtually all depressed people experience sleep disturbance, particularly early-morning awakenings. As a rule the more severe the sleep disorder, the more serious the case of depression, at least as measured on standard psychiatric tests. Generally the depressed sleep less than normal individuals. However, about 15 to 20 percent of depressed people, including adolescents, may sleep more. In severe cases the victim obtains less total sleep and experiences more periods of wakefulness during the night than nondepressed people.

A great deal of research is currently being conducted to study the effects of depression on sleep cycles as detected through EEG tracings. For example, we know now that depressed patients show considerably more Stage 1 (light) sleep but less Stages 3–4 (deep) sleep than normal people. In some specific types of depression there is a shorter period of time, technically known as latency, between the onset of sleep and the first REM period. This reduced REM latency seems to be connected with other symptoms of depression, including loss of appetite, dulled mood, and the absence of pleasurable feelings. The depressive's first REM period is usually long and active, while in normal people the busiest REM period occurs at the end of the night. Depressed people also have more REM episodes. I should point out, however, that it is possible to exhibit the sleep disturbances associated with depression without actually developing other symptoms of the illness. Similarly, impaired sleep continuity and loss of slow-wave sleep are common to many psychiatric disorders, including anxiety, obsessive-compulsive behavior, schizophrenia, and alcoholism.

These sleep abnormalities persist even beyond the period during which a depressed individual experiences symptoms. Eventually, it is thought, the EEG may help physicians refine their diagnosis of depressed patients to differentiate between some of the more subtle forms of the disorder as well as the other psychiatric conditions just noted. Approximately 90 percent of depressives show some form of EEG-verified sleep disturbance. Some experts believe that such clues as REM latency can be used to diagnose past or predict future occurrence of depression in certain patient types.

What's more, study of EEG tracings can help us monitor the way a patient is responding to treatment. Many antidepressant medications serve to suppress REM sleep—in fact, REM suppression may be one of the mechanisms by which such drugs work. (Interestingly, depressed patients also show improvement when they are deprived of REM sleep merely by being awakened at those points in the sleep cycle.) A patient who experiences REM sleep immediately after dropping off is thought to be responding poorly to antidepressants and may need to try a combination of drugs. Similarly, some patients who may respond better to electroshock therapy tend to show much shorter onset of REM sleep than others. Perhaps in the not-too-distant future physicians will be able to diagnose and categorize a patient's illness and prescribe appropriate therapy primarily on the basis of EEG sleep records.

In addition to depression, sleep disturbances are associated with a range of other psychiatric conditions, among them:

* anxiety disorders, in which apprehension and uncertainty become magnified to the point at which they interfere with daily living.

* panic disorder, a form of anxiety characterized by sudden attacks of irrational terror and accompanying feelings of choking, pounding heart, dizziness, and sweating. Unlike patients
  with depression, those with panic disorders who have been
  deprived of a night's sleep are more likely to experience a
  panic attack on the following day.
* phobia, a reaction that is far out of proportion to the actual
  danger present and that interferes with normal functioning.
  Many of us have fears that are rational and reasonable; it is
  appropriate to fear fire, for example, because it can certainly
  hurt or destroy you. A phobia about fire, however, might lead
  a person to become frightened by the sight of a gas stove or
  refuse to enter a building made of wood. A range of phobias,
  from fear of heights to fear of open spaces, has been identified.
* obsessive-compulsive disorders, seen in people who repeatedly
  perform certain acts or rituals. One common example is the
  person whose obsession is cleanliness; the compulsive behavior that results might take the form of washing the hands
  hundreds of times a day.

It is not possible in a book of this nature to describe all of the
therapeutic strategies available for the treatment of these psychiatric disorders. The type of antidepressive medications
known as tricyclics have proven very helpful in cases of depression; some forms of psychosis may respond to an antipyschotic
drug. Sometimes a combination is needed in order to achieve
success. Electroshock therapy may help some depressed patients. In virtually any case, however, psychological counseling
is crucial if the patient is to understand and manage the disorder.

I must emphasize, as I have before, that treating the insomniac component of these disorders without taking the whole complex of symptoms into account is not only unproductive but possibly dangerous as well. Use of a sleeping pill to achieve sleep
may make the patient feel more rested temporarily but does
nothing to penetrate and manage the larger psychiatric disorder. Only when the physician addresses the underlying problem will the insomnia be conquered on any but a short-term
basis.

Abuse of Drugs and Alcohol

Earlier (see page 48–51) I discussed ways that alcohol and illegal drugs such as marijuana and cocaine can contribute to problems of initiating and maintaining sleep. Many other drugs used to treat a variety of medical conditions also possess the undesirable side effect of disturbed sleep. Barbiturates and other hypnotic drugs, for example, may produce sleep disruptions not only while they are being used but during the period of withdrawal as well. Some benzodiazepines have a short half-life (the period in which half the drug is metabolized), in some cases as little as four hours. This is desirable when control must be exercised over how long the drug acts in the body; the downside is that once the drug begins to wear off, sleeplessness may return. This phenomenon is called rebound insomnia. Interrupted sleep is also associated with the use of or withdrawal from those agents used in cancer chemotherapy and thyroid preparations, opiates, and anticonvulsive drugs.

Often a patient is reluctant to tell me about the use of controlled substances, especially the illegal ones or stimulants such as amphetamines. If I suspect that is the case, I will order blood or urine analysis tests. In extreme cases the use of EEG tracings can indicate the presence of drugs. My interest in ordering such tests is not to catch a patient in the act but to obtain as complete a medical profile as possible, so that I can understand the true nature of the problem and deal with it in the most appropriate fashion.

Breathing Disorders

Respiratory ailments such as sleep apnea are notorious for their role in disturbing sleep. There are two primary types of sleep apnea: *obstructive,* in which the airways become blocked for one of a number of reasons, and *central,* in which the physiological mechanisms controlling breathing are disrupted. Sometimes the apnea is a result of both types, and is thus known as *mixed apnea.* At this point I will briefly discuss those breathing disorders that are specifically associated with DIMS; for the most part these fall into the central sleep apnea category (CSA). However, I want to point out that obstructive sleep apnea (OSA) is a more common problem. Like CSA, OSA can occasionally result in the disorders of maintaining sleep that are the focus of this chapter; more often, however, OSA is manifested as a disorder of excessive sleepiness (DOES) and as such will be covered in greater detail in Chapter 6.

Relatively little is known about central sleep apnea. In CSA something—perhaps disruptions in circadian cycles, perhaps some facet of the sleep process itself—causes perturbations in the basic system that drives your breathing cycle. As a result you may cease to breathe temporarily, or your breathing may become too infrequent or too shallow to provide adequate oxygenation of the blood and tissues. As described earlier, your brain will then alert you to awaken in order to overcome the problem. Normally we awaken several times a night anyway, usually at the end of a REM period. With central apnea, however, the arousals are frequent and prevent you from enjoying a good night's sleep.

Other specific forms of CSA include alveolar hypoventilation, which occurs during sleep when the breathing rate or the amount of air inhaled decreases. In some cases hypoventilation is a result of obesity; excess body weight prevents the lungs from expanding to their full capacity. In other patients the problem may be related to specific disorders of the muscles, nerves, or bones, or it may be due to some basic malfunctioning of the respiratory centers located in the brain stem. Yet another variety of CSA is Cheyne-Stokes breathing, the name given to the dyspnea (breathing difficulty) that afflicts patients with left ventricular failure. When heart failure occurs, possibly as a result of some disruption in the nerves, circulation is slowed, the oxygen level of the blood drops, and the level of acids and other toxins increases, giving rise to alternating periods of apnea (breathing cessation) and hyperpnea (gasping, panting breathing).

Victims of CSA are often unaware that the problem exists, because they breathe normally during the day. One clue may be that the patient snores at night; generally, however, snoring is more likely to be a symptom of obstructive apnea. CSA is usually worst during REM sleep because the system that responds to elevated levels of carbon dioxide in the blood is suspended during

REM sleep. Consequently, interruptions in breathing last longer, and the level of oxygen falls to a lower point than during NREM stages. Alcohol, which suppresses the central respiratory drive, only makes the problem worse. Patients with heart disease may experience arrhythmias or increased blood pressure, although these risks are even greater in cases of OSA.

As I mentioned, obstructive sleep apnea may also lead to a DIMS problem, especially if patients become aware that they suffer from the disorder. This often happens if they remember that they have awakened frequently, or if their bed partners have told them about their snoring. If these patients begin to worry about their impaired breathing, they may develop a fear of falling asleep and thus induce a kind of secondary insomnia by forcing themselves to stay awake as long as possible. Therapy for such a problem must be twofold: the cause of the obstructed breathing needs to be discovered and managed, and the psychophysiologic pattern of behavior must be thwarted before it becomes entrenched. Details on the management of OSA also appear in Chapter 6.

Management of CSA usually involves the use of drugs, such as protriptyline, imipramine, or aminophylline, which are known to stimulate the breathing drive. Weight loss is also necessary in obese individuals. Sometimes an electric pacemaker designed to stimulate the diaphragm works in cases where the disordered breathing poses a threat to life. Unfortunately, such pacing cannot be timed to synchronize with the natural breathing rhythm; consequently obstructive apnea may develop, requiring separate treatment. For those patients in whom Cheyne-Stokes breathing produces severely lowered oxygen levels, a drug called acetazolamide sodium has some benefits. The rate of success with all of these therapies, however, is somewhat low.

Restless Legs

Another way your sleep can be disturbed is through pain, discomfort, or twitching in the legs. One form of this condition bears the nontechnical name "restless legs syndrome." If you are a victim of the syndrome, you experience a disagreeable sensation in the calves and feet. Some patients describe twitching or a feeling of "creepy crawling" in the skin, which causes an almost uncontrollable urge to move the legs by walking or shaking or massaging them. This feeling tends to occur during the process of falling asleep, and thus delaying sleep onset; in some cases, however, it can start later and awaken you, forcing you to leave your bed and walk around. Restless legs can be an inherited condition; it may also arise as a complication of pregnancy.

There are drugs that may help the problem: for years doctors in England have treated leg cramps (which they aptly call "the fidgets") with quinine sulfate. Some physicians detect improvement after administering preparations containing all of the B vitamins. Others report success using temazepam (Restoril) or a drug called carbamazepine (sold as Tegretol).

Nighttime Muscle-Twitching

Restless legs syndrome is different from another condition called nocturnal myoclonus, which means "nighttime muscle-twitching" and is the name given to the problem of frequent strong leg jerks. Sleep laboratory studies have found that some patients may have leg jerks three hundred to four hundred times a night, occurring every twenty to forty seconds. Both legs are usually involved. Unlike restless legs syndrome, myocolonus causes no unpleasant sensations in the leg. Because it occurs during sleep, episodes are seldom recalled. Myoclonus may arise from such medical problems as kidney disease, metabolic disorders, narcolepsy, drug withdrawal, or apnea. Withdrawal from medications, such as antidepressants or anticonvulsive drugs, can serve to worsen the problem. I should stress that myoclonus is not a seizure disorder like epilepsy. EEG tracings of people with myoclonus indicate that both their sleep and their waking patterns are normal (except for the nighttime arousals caused by twitching).

Obviously, victims of myoclonus have trouble maintaining sleep. While they may not actually awaken during a twitching episode, these patients may perceive their sleep to be light, broken, and restless. They may also awaken feeling unrested and unrestored. Frequently, too, their bed partners complain of disturbed sleep, pointing to the bruises on their shins as evidence. Researchers estimate that as many as 10 to 15 percent of patients with a sleep disorder have nocturnal myoclonus; an estimated one out of three people over the age of sixty-five are thought to suffer from the problem. The drug temazepam may provide relief; if after a few weeks the problem persists, some physicians may decide to prescribe a drug called clonazepam (marketed as Klonopin). No one is certain if clonazepam works because it relaxes leg muscles or because it possesses anticonvulsive properties.

Medical Causes of DIMS

In Chapter 2 I discussed the many medical conditions that may lead to disturbed sleep. Briefly, then, let me reiterate that such problems as chronic pain, arthritis, hyperthyroidism, heartburn, or breathing conditions such as cough or COPD can cause DIMS. Sometimes the drugs used to treat these conditions can disrupt sleep, either because they stimulate the system, as do beta-adrenergic agonists or steroids, or because they have a rebound effect when the medication wears off. More rarely hypothyroidism or some abnormal tissue growths may affect the central respiratory drive.

Childhood DIMS

Another category of DIMS encompasses those sleep problems that begin during childhood or before puberty and persist into adulthood. While largely similar to the psychophysiological DIMS I described earlier, these childhood-onset disorders lack discernible conditioning factors, arising instead out of early emotional turmoil or psychiatric disturbance. One distinguishing factor of these sleep problems is that they remain relatively constant over time, regardless of the emotional arousal experienced by the individual. Such sleep disorders are notoriously resistant to treatment, because they may stem from malfunctions of the central nervous system that have existed since birth.

Sleep-Cycle Disruptions

Sometimes DIMS may arise from some kind of ingrained disturbance in the sleep pattern. For example, you may experience awakening during your first nightly REM sleep period, then continue to awaken during as much as 75 to 100 percent of the remaining REM time throughout the night, finding it difficult or impossible to return to sleep. If so, you may be losing as much as four to six hours of rest a night. REM-interruption insomnia is more common in men, especially after the age of thirty-five, and has been linked to emotional disturbance and, as we have seen, to depression.

EEG tracings indicate that the REM-period awakenings follow a burst of intense eye movement, perhaps caused by the onset of a dream. It might seem logical to conclude that the dream itself prompts the awakening, but research does not really support this idea. Actually, you may find you experience REM interruptions if at some point in the past, perhaps a time of emotional trouble, you have suffered a nightmare or even a series of nightmares. As a result your intrinsic sleep control mechanism may have become programmed to awaken you before or as dreams occur, in a well-meaning but ultimately harmful effort to avoid nightmares by preventing the onset of REM sleep. It is harmful because, as we have seen, REM deprivation may aggravate other psychotic symptoms. In a sense, then, REM interruptions are a kind of conditioned-response DIMS.

Another sleep-pattern disturbance is identified on EEG tracings as the presence of alpha waves during the NREM phases of the cycle, which indicates that the brain experiences waking activity even while it is supposedly asleep. Alpha waves are not usually recorded during REM sleep. Not surprisingly, sleep that is riddled with alpha waves is interrupted and nonrestorative. Victims will awaken feeling tired and unrested and will often underestimate the amount of sleep they actually obtained; they describe their nights as marked by a "sense of continued vigilance." Withdrawal from alcohol and some drugs may result in the superimposition of alpha waves onto the normal sleep pattern.

Short Sleepers

Most forms of DIMS fall into one or another of the categories I've just described; occasionally, however, I will run across cases that fit none of them. There is no doubt that the patients suffer from insomnia—they sleep less than they feel is right for them.

But when I examine them I am unable to discern any physical or psychological abnormality. Even the results of a sleep lab study may demonstrate no objective findings, by any of the usual clinical measurements, to indicate that sleep was disturbed, yet the patients insist that sleep was somehow unsatisfactory. Such patients are known as "short sleepers," meaning that their sleep lasts less than 75 percent of the time considered average for their age group. Any symptoms they experience as a result of their sleep patterns are not directly related to their perceived insomnia. Rather, problems arise from their basic concern that they are somehow "abnormal," that they should be sleeping differently from how they are. Sometimes these patients express the belief that there is a certain amount of sleep they "should" be getting—what I call the eight-hour myth. They may also feel lonely because they are awake during the early hours of the morning, or because there is relatively little support from our culture for people who do not fit the normal pattern of rest and waking. One short-sleeper acquaintance told me she would wake up hours before she had to be at work and do nothing except worry about her job. By the time she got there she was a nervous wreck. However, her life and her work improved tremendously when she began an early-morning hobby: writing. She is now writing a sequel to her first, unpublished spy novel.

Often a patient's description of a sleep problem may initially suggest a disorder in initiating or maintaining sleep. As I've mentioned, however, careful attention to the patient's sleep patterns, drug use, and medical history may help further differentiate the true nature of the disorder. Sometimes reassessment is mandated when the initial approach to therapy is insufficient or completely unsuccessful. If so, the diagnosis may be changed to one of the other categories of insomnia, such as DOES, which will be covered in the next chapter.

6

Why You Can't Stay Awake

The previous chapter focused on the problems that can prevent you from falling asleep or that cause you to awaken during the night. Let's look now at a category that is actually more common: the disorders of excessive sleepiness (DOES), also known as hypersomnia.

Naturally we have all experienced days when, for one reason or another, we simply cannot—or will not—drag ourselves out of bed. According to writer Anthony Burgess, our understandable reluctance to rise may be nothing more than a recollection of "the perfectly tempered warmth of the womb; the cold out there is more than a matter of temperature, it is an aspect of the iron hardness of the cruel world." If we do manage to extract ourselves from the bed, we proceed to stagger through our daily routines, barely aware of our surroundings, unable to keep our eyes open or our mind focused. We may doze off at our desk or, even worse, behind the wheel of a car. Such periods of occasional somnolence are normal, arising from temporary disruptions in our daily schedule or a transient perturbation in our circadian rhythms.

A disorder of excessive sleepiness, on the other hand, is more serious; such a disorder is a medical problem which persists over time and interferes with everyday living. By sleepiness I mean simply that the patient perceives the need to sleep. Victims of DOES—15 percent of the population by some estimates—may describe themselves as constantly sleepy, or they may be subject to periodic attacks of sleepiness, or both. For some, although they are able to function to one degree or another, there is a constant battle to stay awake. For others, the desire to sleep is so overwhelming that they are forced to nap, often at inappropriate times. DOES victims may experience such effects as decreased cognitive and motor functioning, fatigue, depression, and an increase in time spent asleep over a twenty-four-hour period.

Patients have described their condition to me in many ways. One man stated, "I have absolutely no energy; sometimes I feel I can barely hold my head up. My boss thinks I'm bored in my job—I'm not. I love my work. But sometimes I just want to curl up on the floor of the office and snooze for the rest of the afternoon." Another said he was so groggy on rising that he thought he had been drinking the night before, to the point where he couldn't remember whether he'd drunk or not. A woman said she felt "weary all the time, no matter how much sleep I got the night before." She assumed she was clinically depressed, because she felt an overpowering urge to crawl into bed and pull the covers over her head. One patient was terrified by the overpowering attacks of sleepiness and muscle paralysis he experienced during moments of emotional arousal. In addition to feeling weary or exhausted, victims of DOES may claim that their sleep is nonrestorative, light, or fragmented. As one patient said, "My batteries just never seem to get recharged the way they used to." Obviously, these problems, left untreated, can interfere with social, work, and family obligations.

Excessive daytime sleepiness is the major complaint of those people who seek help from sleep-disorder clinics. In one study, 51 percent of patients were diagnosed as suffering from hypersomnia, while 31 percent suffered one of the forms of insomnia described earlier. Each year, sleep-disorder centers report seeing as many as 30,000 new patients with some form of DOES complaint.

Statistically, most cases of daytime sleepiness arise from disordered breathing during the night—the sleep apnea I described briefly in the previous chapter, in the context of sleep interruption. According to one study, as many as 43 percent of DOES victims have a breathing abnormality, primarily of the obstructive variety. During the night, these patients experience stoppages of breath lasting 20, 40, even 90 seconds, which in turn cause them to waken to some degree or another. Come morning, apneics feel unrested and lethargic; surprisingly, however, many of them have no idea that their breathing at night is abnormal, since during the day they experience no breathing difficulty. We will take a closer look at sleep apnea, including the condition known as sudden infant death syndrome, shortly.

The next most frequent cause of hypersomnia is narcolepsy. Victims of this strange disorder do not necessarily feel tired during the day; however, they are frequently overwhelmed by sudden, uncontrollable attacks of sleepiness. One of the most prominent—and troubling—features of narcolepsy is cataplexy, or muscle paralysis, a symptom that distinguishes this condition from other forms of hypersomnia. Narcolepsy accounts for roughly one-fourth of all DOES diagnoses. In fact, seven out of ten patients who are seen by sleep laboratories are diagnosed as having either sleep apnea or narcolepsy.

Less frequently, DOES may be the result of nocturnal myoclonus if the leg jerks are powerful enough to cause partial arousal during sleep. Like apneics, victims of myoclonus may be unaware their sleep has been disrupted, noticing only that they are still tired the following the day. Other sources of daytime sleepiness include psychiatric disorders such as depression, use and abuse of drugs or alcohol, and a whole range of metabolic, endocrine, and central nervous system disorders. When we are unable to identify a specific cause for hypersomnia, we classify it as "idiopathic," which means "caused by itself" or "of unknown origin." Nearly one out of ten cases of DOES fits this vague but convenient category. I will also devote part of this chapter to a discussion of another variety of sleep problem, disorders of the sleep-wake schedule (DSWS) which, though of a different nature from DOES, can also produce the symptom of daytime sleepiness.

As we will see, diagnosis of DOES can be tricky. Daytime tiredness can mask a number of other problems, including drug use, poor nutrition, emotional frustration, dissatisfaction, or poor motivation. Many forms of psychological disruption can sap our energy, disturb our rest, and exhaust us even more than strenuous physical activity. Lifestyle can contribute as well: if you lead a sedentary life, for example, you omit the exercise that gives the body the chance to purge itself of waste products and restore energy to the muscles.

As a doctor, my challenge is to distinguish true cases of hypersomnia from the chronic, low-level fatigue and tiredness that sometimes afflict people who, while basically normal, may be bored, restless, or otherwise unhappy. I must also sort out those patients who are simply unaware that they are not getting enough sleep to meet their daytime needs. Often these are people who hold two jobs, or who cram their days so full of activities that they do not allow sufficient time for sleep. Yet another type of patient excluded from the DOES category is the "healthy hypersomniac," the person who simply needs more sleep than other people—possibly as many as fourteen hours. These long sleepers may not complain of excessive sleepiness, but, like their short-sleeping counterparts discussed in the previous chapter, they may experience some kind of psychological fallout if they think of themselves as abnormal or experience social isolation as a result of their sleep patterns.

Among the questions I might ask you to determine if DOES is a problem in your case: is your feeling of sleepiness constant, or does it appear only at certain times? When do episodes of sleepiness occur? In what ways does the sleepiness affect you: do you take naps, for example, or struggle constantly to stay awake? How well do you function generally during the day? I would also conduct a number of clinical tests in order to rule out such causes of excessive sleepiness as hypothyroidism, hypoglycemia, drug abuse, metabolic disorders, even brain tumor. If none of these pathologies could be identified, then I would be reasonably certain you had a true disorder of excessive sleepiness.

SLEEP APNEA

As we have seen, sleep apnea is an interval of interrupted or arrested breathing followed by loud gasping, choking, or snoring, which may result in partial or full arousal. The victim struggles to regain breath, sometimes with a great heaving of the chest. While the heaving, often desperate breathing pattern of an apnea victim does serve to restore airflow, it can actually aggravate the condition. Trying to breathe against the "gag" reflex creates abnormal air pressure in the passageways and can impair blood flow. Consequently the blood pressure rises as the heart beats irregularly, sometimes almost frantically. When the victim finally does breathe again, the massive inrush of air into the lungs produces a loud choking gasp or snore. You can easily see the effect for yourself: try inhaling while consciously blocking off the intake of air by preventing it from passing through your throat. Then, while still trying to inhale, suddenly relax your throat—and notice the impact.

Sleep apnea, as noted earlier, is classified as *central* (if the cause stems from a disorder affecting the central respiratory drive) or *obstructive* (if a physical defect leads to blocked airways). The more sleep researchers learn about these conditions, however, the more the distinctions between them become blurred. "Pure" central sleep apnea (CSA)—the total absence of breathing effort and airflow through the nose and mouth—and "pure" obstructive sleep apnea (OSA)—decreased or absent airflow coupled with increased breathing effort—are rarely seen. More often the problem is a mixture of the two: a central malfunction that in turn causes some kind of airway blockage. CSA was discussed in the previous chapter because it often results in nighttime awakenings. Here we will focus on OSA because of its association with excessive daytime sleepiness.

To be considered clinically significant, the lack of airflow must last for at least ten seconds; some reports describe patients who stop breathing for up to a minute and a half. (For some reason, you are able to hold your breath longer when you are asleep than when you are awake.) Normally everyone experiences four or five apneic episodes per hour of sleep, but patients with sleep-disordered breathing may have five hundred, eight hundred, even a thousand episodes in an eight-hour period. People who experience a thousand microarousals over the course of a night—an average of one every thirty seconds—understandably feel, on rising, that they didn't sleep at all. However, unless these victims have been aroused for ten to fifteen seconds, they are not likely to realize that their sleep has been disturbed. Consequently they may wonder why they feel sleepy during the day.

Who Suffers From Sleep Apnea?

Surprisingly, sleep apnea was not identified as a diagnosable condition until the early 1970s. Now, however, it is ranked as the single most frequent cause of sleep disturbance, occurring in almost half of patients with sleeping problems. Overall perhaps 5 percent of the U.S. population—roughly 12 million people—may suffer from it. One out of ten men over forty have clinically significant sleep apnea. The older you are, the greater the risk: some experts estimate that 40 to 50 percent of the population over the age of fifty may experience sleep-disordered breathing.

The pattern of daytime sleepiness resulting from apnea varies widely. Some people with OSA are prone to sleep attacks and microsleeps—dozings that last only a second or two. Usually they find naps do little to refresh them. Like narcoleptics, they may experience hallucinations as they wake up or drop off, but they don't exhibit the telltale narcolepsy symptom of muscle paralysis. Other OSA victims fall asleep whenever their activity level drops below a certain point—when they sit down, for example, or as soon as they begin to read. Driving is a notorious trigger for sleepiness; one patient described himself as "catnapping on the straightaways and waking up for the curves." Sufferers may have lower levels of attention and concentration and have been found less able to perform small manipulations with their hands, such as knitting or typing. In severe cases OSA can make it impossible for a person to function on the job; many a patient, like the one I mentioned earlier, has told me of stern reprimands or even firings by unsympathetic bosses. Diagnosis is often made more difficult by patients who deny the severity of the problem.

The Physical Causes of Sleep Apnea

What is the physical process that leads to sleep apnea? Almost always apneic episodes result from an obstruction of the pharynx occurring somewhere between the nose and the epiglottis—

the membrane that prevents food from going down the wrong "pipe." The upper airway, from the mouth and nose to the lungs, is not just a hollow tube through which breath moves: the coordinated activity of a number of muscles is required if this airway is to work efficiently and effectively. As we breathe in, these muscles must contract, in synchronized fashion, to pull the passage open: this muscle contraction, as well as our instinct to breathe, is controlled by the central respiratory drive in the brain. Like many bodily structures, the upper airway is pretty delicate: it doesn't take a very big difference in air pressure between the atmosphere and the inside of the throat to cause the passageway to collapse. The muscles must therefore work continually to keep the tube open.

As we have seen, a number of factors—among them drugs, alcohol, and, to some extent, sleep itself—can suppress the central respiratory drive, especially during slow-wave sleep and the REM phase. Alcohol is a particular threat; not only does it suppress the breathing drive, it also relaxes the throat muscles, reducing their ability to keep the airway open. What's more, alcohol weakens the mechanism that helps us wake up quickly, thus adding to the time it takes to become aroused enough to make the conscious effort needed to breathe. I tell all patients with apnea that use of alcohol, other than perhaps a very small quantity (less than an ounce), is inadvisable. If they must drink, I ask them to do so no later than four to six hours before bedtime.

In addition to suppressed respiratory drive, another factor in apnea is the horizontal position we assume during sleep, which can lead to narrowing of the air passage. The breathing tube collapses somewhat because of the weight of the body pressing down from above, and it is further obstructed to a degree because the tongue moves from its usual waking position to a position farther back in the throat. Also, during the night the coughing mechanism is somewhat suppressed, and the lungs are less able to clear themselves of secretions. All of these slowdowns in breathing function are normal and pose no threat to the majority of people. When complicated by other factors, however, they can result in OSA.

Results of the physical examination of an apnea victim are often relatively normal. I may, and often do, find elevated blood pressure, or I may notice that the mouth and pharynx are smaller than normal or "crowded" due to some kind of unusual structural formation. On listening to the neck I may hear stridor—the harsh, high-pitched sound associated with obstruction of the larynx. In cases where the heart has been affected, I may detect signs of right ventricular failure, such as distension of the jugular vein or swelling of the ankles. Analysis of gasses in the blood may reveal a high level of carbon dioxide; if so, I will want to rule out some other form of lung disease by ordering further pulmonary tests.

There are a number of physical problems that can also provide hints about the causes of a patient's OSA. As you might expect, if you are overweight you are more prone to airway obstruction. Your respiratory muscles may be unable to overcome the additional pressure from body weight in order to contract and keep the airway open. Furthermore, accumulations of fatty tissue in this region of the body may act to block the passage of air. Sleep apnea is especially common in children with large tonsils and adenoids. If obesity is also present, these children are known by the rather unflattering sobriquet "chubby puffers."

Apnea can also arise from an excessively thick palate, an enlarged uvula or thyroid gland, or such deformities as retrognathia (receding jaw), micrognathia (small jaw), or bony abnormalities of the upper airway, including a short neck, which can position the tongue too close to the back of the pharyngeal wall and thus reduce airflow. Conditions such as amyloidosis (accumulation of starchy substance in tissue) or myxedema (swelling associated with hypothyroidism) can result in an enlarged tongue, causing obstructed breathing. Hypothyroidism blunts the respiratory drive and may also contribute to obesity. Sometimes lesions in the nose can be a factor in collapse of the airways, and polyps or tumors in the larynx can also lead to apnea. Acromegaly, an oversecretion of growth hormone that causes enlargements in skeletal extremities, including the jaw and nose, can do so as well.

On more than one occasion I've seen a patient whose dentures were to blame: badly fitting false teeth can cause the muscles of the mouth to strain to keep them in place. Removing the dentures at night can lead to unusual relaxation of the muscles, in turn causing the airways in the mouth and throat to collapse to some degree.

Sometimes, in rare cases, the cause is more serious—pharyngeal cancer, for example, or a neurological disease such as poliomyelitis, myasthenia gravis (a disease that can produce fatigue in the muscle systems of the throat and neck), or amyotrophic lateral sclerosis (an often fatal degeneration of the brain stem and spinal cord). In other cases, spinal surgery, brain stem infarction or growth, pulmonary disease, or cardiac disorders may be responsible.

The Dangers of Sleep Apnea

Sleep apnea poses a number of health risks, ranging from mild to life-threatening. Among these:

High Blood Pressure When breathing stops, the brain signals the heart to pump more vigorously to compensate for the drop in oxygen supply. Blood pressure thus rises sharply; in severe cases, this increase can lead to cardiac arrest, which can be fatal.

One study found that patients with sleep apnea were five times as likely to have high blood pressure as those who were unaffected by nighttime breathing disturbance. Between 60 and 80 percent of patients with OSA also have hypertension. Also, about 30 percent of patients with hypertension suffer from OSA—a significantly higher incidence of OSA than that found in the general population, which is estimated to be 5 percent. Such results indicate that OSA plays a direct role in elevating blood pressure. The same study found that hypertensive patients had an average of 110 apneic episodes per night, compared with 11 experienced by nonhypertensive individuals. There are two conclusions to be drawn from such data: if you have hypertension, it should be treated in order to minimize the risk of OSA (and for many other reasons as well). Conversely, if you have OSA, it should be treated to lower the risk of developing a chronic case of high blood pressure.

Other Cardiac Complications Apnea has been shown to lead to chronic heart disease or cardiopulmonary failure, causing a buildup of toxins and acids in the blood. Hypoxemia (lowered oxygen), which results in lowered cardiac output, increases the risk of strokes or myocardial ischemia. It may also generate one or more types of irregular heartbeats, some of which can be lethal. Incidence of some heart problems is at its highest during the early-morning hours, a phenomenon which many experts feel is related to breathing disturbances during sleep. OSA is thought to be responsible for as many as two to three thousand cases each year of sudden death during sleep.

Other Risks Lowered blood output means that less blood, and thus less oxygen, is circulated to the brain. Naturally this has a detrimental effect on brain-stem functioning; the brain becomes less able to work at overcoming the problem of disordered breathing, thus causing further hypoxemia. Unless this vicious circle is broken, the apneas will become more frequent and pro-longed, and symptoms will worsen, starting with restless sleep and excessive daytime sleepiness and eventually progressing to stupor or even coma. Apnea may also contribute to the decline of mental functioning associated with aging, resulting in loss of memory, diminished attention span, confusion, and impaired cognitive and motor performance. Some patients report changes in personality, including irritability and mood swings. In some cases apnea leads to problems of impotence, diminished sex drive, bed-wetting, and, in men, difficulty with erection and ejac-ulation.

Sickle-cell anemia poses a special risk for OSA victims, since lowered oxygen saturation at night can precipitate an anemic crisis. Similarly, polycythemia—elevation of the total red cell mass—may occur due to episodes of apnea resulting in lowered oxygen in the arteries.

SNORING

Snoring, of course, is the most prominent symptom of sleep apnea. I want to make it clear, however, that snoring and OSA are not synonymous. While virtually all OSA patients snore—long and loud—not everyone who snores has a clinically signifi-cant OSA problem.

People who snore have been the targets of humor, and anger, for centuries. And no wonder: *The Guinness Book of World Rec-ords* has clocked the loudest snore at 87.5 decibels—equivalent to the noise of a bus's diesel engine heard from the rear seat or the sound of a pneumatic drill as it breaks up concrete. Not infrequently snoring is cited as one reason a married couple seeks a divorce.

Among people aged thirty to thirty-five, 20 percent of men but only 5 percent of women snore. As age increases, however, so does the incidence of snoring. Half of the population over the age of forty snores. Most of this group is still men, but by age sixty the split is closer to 60–40. By age sixty-five the division is roughly even, with as many as 6 to 7 million elderly Americans snoring away through the night. Science has proposed no sound theory (excuse the pun) to explain why there is a difference in the incidence of snoring between younger men and women. However, it is abundantly clear that obesity makes a difference: snoring is three times more common in obese individuals of both sexes.

Anybody can snore—great and near great, famous and infamous. Among the American presidents who shook the walls of the White House were Adams (both of them), Van Buren, Fillmore, Pierce, Buchanan, Lincoln, Andrew Johnson, Grant, Hayes, Arthur, Cleveland, Harrison, McKinley, Roosevelt (both of them), Taft, Harding, and Hoover. (Washington snored too, but he never lived in the White House.) Teddy Roosevelt once so disturbed the hospital where he was being treated that nearly every patient in the wing filed a complaint. Other historical noisemakers include Emperor Otho, Cato, King George (II and IV), Lord Chesterfield, Beau Brummel, Winston Churchill, and Benito Mussolini. And although snoring is rarely fatal, the nineteenth-century gunman John Wesley Hardin is reported to have been so annoyed by the noise generated by a guest sleeping in the same hotel that he went into the room and shot him to death.

One patient told me his wife complained that she couldn't hear the phone when he snored. Another was referred for treatment because his wife, a musician, couldn't bear his off-pitch nocturnes. In Cincinnati a man who had been sentenced to three months in jail was released after only a few days; the other prisoners complained that his snoring constituted cruel and unusual punishment, and the warden agreed.

(And humans are not the only players in this nighttime symphony. Among the animals who have been found to snore are buffaloes, camels, cats, chimpanzees, cows, dogs, elands, elephants, gorillas, horses, leopards, mules, oxen, sheep, tigers, and zebras.)

One writer, motivated by complaints about his own nighttime noise, researched the topic and devised a classification system identifying eleven different types of snoring, to which he gave the names laryngeal, nasal, obesial, neurotic, pathologic, physiologic, functional, lateral, supine, prone, and pseudosnoring— noise which is made to add verisimilitude to the pretense of sleep. I must confess, however, I find that most of these labels fall far short of having any practical value in the management of sleep apnea.

Common "Cures" for Snoring

Folklore is replete with suggestions on how to curb snoring, including sleeping on a wooden pillow, as do the Japanese, or having someone whistle near the snorer's ear. One suggestion frequently proposed is to sew a tennis ball or some other object into the pajamas in order to prevent snorers from sleeping on their backs. Nearly two hundred antisnoring devices have been patented in a vain effort to squelch the problem. These inventions—mostly commercial variations on old folk remedies— range from mouth gags, muzzles, and chin straps to nasal tubes and neck collars to prevent the neck from kinking. Other, somewhat more elaborate methods which have been tried (and have largely failed) include amputation of the uvula (a small fleshy extension of the soft palate, just above the root of the tongue), which was standard operating procedure a century ago, and injection of paraffin or some other hardening agent into the soft palate to make it resistant to vibration.

Antisnoring Tips

If obstructive apnea is the cause of snoring, the only real long-term hope is to find and manage the immediate cause. For example, surgery can correct the deviated septum often blamed for snoring. I'll describe other medical remedies for OSA shortly (see page 133). In the meantime, if you or your spouse snore, some nonmedical techniques may supply a degree of relief.

* Sleep with more than one pillow, so as to keep the head elevated.
* Tuck tiny balls of tissue into the pocket of each nostril at the tip of the nose, to keep the nostrils open and direct airflow to minimize vibration of the soft palate.
* If you wear dentures, try keeping them in at night.
* Let the nonsnorer go to bed earlier.
* If necessary, sleep in different beds or bedrooms.
* If all else fails, the nonsnorer should try earplugs.

Management of Apnea

As we saw in the previous chapter, the options for drug therapy in the treatment of sleep apnea are few and relatively ineffective. Some drugs may be appropriate when central apnea is the problem, since they act to repair the mechanisms responsible for a malfunctioning respiratory drive. Protriptyline, for example, stimulates the muscles of the upper airway; it also decreases the time spent in REM sleep, thus minimizing the periods during which most severe OSA occurs. In OSA, however, the causes of the breathing disruption are usually of a physical nature, making drug therapy largely useless. Sleeping pills, commercial or prescription, are no solution. I have discussed the fact that use of sedatives may produce sleep but can also act to prevent the sleeper from waking up enough to begin breathing after an apnea attack. What's more, such drugs suppress respiratory function even further—in some cases to the point of death.

By the same token, however, to delay treatment, or avoid it entirely, may be just as dangerous. Besides the health risks posed by apnea, such as hypertension and heart disease, there is the documented danger of death directly attributable to breathing problems.

There are options, however, which can provide varying measures of success but, like almost any medical treatment, have their share of drawbacks as well. As we have seen, most apnea is really a mixture of CSA and OSA. Thus the discussion of treatments here will focus on the latter, since in many cases remedying the obstruction will subsequently eliminate the cause of central apnea as well.

Suppose you come to me as an apneic patient. My first step is to eliminate any agent that may be contributing to your problem—specifically, sedative drugs, hypnotic drugs, or alcohol. Since smoking can also contribute, I'll ask you to stop. If obesity is a factor, I will encourage you to lose weight (unless you have heart arrhythmias or hypoxemia). In many cases weight loss alone helps more than anything else; studies have found that even small amounts of weight loss can improve the oxygenation of the blood and reduce the incidence of daytime sleepiness. In one group of patients who weighed an average of 234 pounds, loss of 22 pounds caused the patients' disordered breathing and daytime symptoms to disappear. Effective weight reduction, however, is very difficult unless you are highly motivated; toward that end I will arrange for adequate supportive therapy. If you are of normal weight, I may suggest ways to vary your sleeping position as the night progresses. Studies show that patients who sleep on their backs have twice as many apnea attacks as those who sleep on their sides.

If the problem continues, and I am unable to spot the cause, I will probably refer you for analysis by a sleep laboratory, a process described later in this book. Depending on the clinical findings, a number of therapeutic options may be called into play. Some of the following options are remedial, not curative; that is to say, they improve your condition without eliminating it.

Continuous Positive Airway Pressure, or CPAP During CPAP you wear a nasal mask attached to a machine that pumps air and provides a constant degree of background pressure in the airway. This pressure keeps the passage between the mouth and the lower pharynx open. CPAP is widely available commercially, reasonably inexpensive (compared to surgery), and relatively simple to operate. But, as one sleep researcher put it, "you have to sleep with a machine that sounds like a vacuum cleaner for the rest of your life." CPAP can be uncomfortable and irritating; in some cases eye complications, stemming from the presence of the mask, have been reported. The most important drawback, however, is psychosocial. For many of my patients, especially the younger ones and their spouses, the thought of sleeping with a nasal mask and an air compressor every night can be disheartening. In those cases where CPAP is appropriate, the patient must possess the proper mental attitude to use the technique correctly and faithfully.

Tracheostomy In this surgery, an opening is made in the trachea to permit the insertion of a breathing tube which bypasses the obstructed segment of the airway. This approach is considered the "gold standard" against which the effectiveness of other treatments is often measured, especially in cases complicated by life-threatening arrhythmias (irregular heart rhythms). Again, however, there are disadvantages. The tracheostomy tube is permanent; it must be carefully cleaned and maintained, posing hygiene problems. Patients often feel a sense of disapproval from society, including friends, relatives, and co-workers who are uncomfortable in the presence of such a device. Obese patients—a significant proportion of apneics—may experience some mechanical difficulty, especially if their necks are particularly fleshy or layered. The recent trend in medicine is to reserve tracheostomy for only the most serious cases; otherwise, it is often difficult to justify its use.

Uvulopalatopharyngoplasty (UPPP) This polysyllabic mouthful is enough to cause shortness of breath in itself; it means plastic surgery involving the uvula, palate, and pharynx. The procedure, first described in 1981 by a Japanese surgeon, was designed to help patients with obstructions of the soft palate or the oropharynx (the part of the pharynx between the soft palate and the upper edge of the epiglottis; obstructions at the base of the tongue are not affected by the surgery). UPPP was performed on over five thousand Americans in 1983–84 alone. Usually, if you are a candidate for the surgery, you will first undergo a screening using a rapid form of computerized imaging known as cine-CT. This procedure, performed while you sleep, measures your airways and allows experts to detect multiple sites of obstruction. Cine-CT is relatively expensive, about $450 per screening, but many physicians feel it will become the primary method for measuring airway obstruction—at least, in hospitals that can afford to purchase a cine-CT unit (approximately $1.5 million apiece!).

At first UPPP generated considerable enthusiasm among apnea specialists, since it appeared to cure three out of four cases. Subsequent reports, however, posted success rates of only 25 to 50 percent, perhaps because in some cases there is an additional airway narrowing at the level of the tongue, not correctable with UPPP. One benefit is that it does seem to cure many cases of snoring by removing the tissue responsible for the resonation. Complications of UPPP include the rather unpleasant experience of nasal regurgitation—reflux of food through the nose while eating. Fortunately, this annoying side effect lasts for only a few days or weeks after surgery.

The ideal candidate for UPPP is somewhat rare: an athletic male, thirty-five years old, with a long dangling uvula, who suffers from severe snoring. If every UPPP patient matched this description, the success rate would approach 100 percent. On the other hand, the very obese patient who might traditionally have undergone a tracheostomy has only a fifty-fifty chance of being helped by UPPP. Further research is under way to determine if there are other patients who could be helped by this technique.

Other Options In children especially, removing the tonsils and adenoids can often eliminate the apnea problem, although, to be honest, we don't really know why. Surgical correction of a cleft palate or removal of any nasal polyps or tumors may provide relief; such problems, however, are rare. When appropriate, a procedure known as mandibular advancement—jaw rearrangement—can help. Also diaphragmatic pacing (a kind of pacemaker for the lungs) may provide some benefits.

SUDDEN INFANT DEATH SYNDROME

Before leaving the subject of sleep apnea, I want to discuss briefly the problem of sudden infant death syndrome—SIDS, also known as crib death. Each year this tragic affliction strikes as many as 10,000 to 18,000 babies between the ages of one and seven months. The exact cause of SIDS, unfortunately, is not yet known. Many experts believe it is a form of sleep apnea during which the baby, whose central nervous system and respiratory drive are not yet fully developed, may stop breathing long enough to result in death. In some cases the infant is found to have a mild case of upper respiratory tract infection, or some mucus plugging the nose—seemingly a minor problem, until you realize that babies don't learn to breathe through their mouths until the age of four months. Yet most normal infants commonly experience short spells of apnea; we don't yet know how to identify those who may be at greater risk of SIDS so as to intervene and prevent its occurrence.

If you are concerned about your child, some approaches to SIDS management are available: monitors attached to the crib may detect a breathing stoppage; alarms will wake the baby, causing it to begin breathing normally, and will alert others in the house as well. One psychologist reports some success in training infants to react vigorously to a breathing obstruction, such as a light cloth placed over the mouth for a short time.

NARCOLEPSY

After apnea, narcolepsy is the next most frequent cause of excessive daytime sleepiness. People with this disorder are prone to transient, overpowering attacks of sleepiness lasting from a few seconds up to thirty minutes, with the average spell lasting about two minutes. Narcoleptics may have up to two hundred such attacks in a single day, even if they have slept well the night before. During an attack the victim's jaw may grow slack, or the head may drop forward onto the chest. In some cases victims may completely black out, appearing to be asleep or unaware of their actions. In less severe attacks, they are alert but may experience some form of muscle paralysis—their knees may buckle, or they may lose all control over their voluntary muscles. (Some people mistakenly refer to narcolepsy as sleeping sickness. The two are by no means the same: sleeping sickness is a parasitic infection transmitted by insects, including the tsetse fly and the kissing bug. Narcolepsy is also distinguished from seizure disorders like epilepsy in that such symptoms as repetitive movements (lip smacking, for example) and perceived visual auras are rarely present.

The term "narcolepsy" was first used more than a century ago, but its symptoms were not delineated and defined until the

1940s. Today an estimated 250,000 Americans suffer from the condition—more than the number of people afflicted with multiple sclerosis. Although narcolepsy accounts for less than 1 percent of all cases of sleep disorders, sleep laboratories report that narcoleptics make up the second largest group of patients who come to them for help.

Symptoms of Narcolepsy

In addition to daytime sleep attacks, the primary symptoms of narcolepsy include sleep paralysis, hallucinations, and cataplexy. Sleep paralysis—sudden inability to move—occurs at the beginning or the end of sleep and renders immobile virtually every voluntary muscle except those around the eyes. When hallucinations are present, they usually come at the beginning of sleep; they may be vivid, realistic, and sometimes violent.

Cataplexy—an attack of muscle weakness or dysfunction lasting from a few seconds to a few minutes—is one of the most disconcerting features of narcolepsy, largely because of the suddenness with which it appears. An attack can be triggered by almost any form of emotional arousal, from anger to athletic activity to excitement—even the mere anticipation of excitement. A mother of three told me she had to allow her children to run amok; she was unable to discipline them because doing so would trigger an attack. Another patient reported that his fraternity brothers considered it an evening's entertainment to regale him with jokes, just to get him to laugh so that they could watch him collapse. Another described his sadness at having to stay away from Yankees baseball games. During any thrilling moment, he said, just as the other fans were rising to their feet, he would crumple to the floor of the stands. In one case reported in the literature a patient became cataplectic every time he had an orgasm. He had naturally come to believe that such paralysis was simply part of the sexual experience. Sometimes the consequences can be disastrous. A narcoleptic butcher fell asleep while wielding a meat cleaver and awakened to find he had lopped off three of his fingers.

Cataplexy may involve all of the muscles or just a select few; the severity ranges from a slight loss of tone to complete paralysis. Victims do not lose consciousness. Not all narcoleptics experience cataplexy; in some, however, the attacks are frequent. People with narcolepsy may notice excessive daytime sleepiness as much as a year before the onset of cataplexy.

Memory difficulties are also reported by about half of narcoleptics. In addition, some experience symptoms in the eyes: fatigue, difficulty focusing, double vision. Except for cataplexy, however, these symptoms are not unique to narcolepsy but are found in other disorders as well.

Possible Causes of Narcolepsy

Usually the onset of narcolepsy occurs during childhood or adolescence. Narcolepsy is thought to arise from some kind of biochemical imbalance or defect in the central nervous system, one that seems to affect the mechanism that activates the "on/ off" cycle of sleep. It is not contagious, but those who report a family history of the disorder are 60 percent more likely to develop it than other people.

By studying the EEG tracings of narcoleptics, researchers have learned that victims are unable to keep the REM phase of the sleep cycle in its proper place. Instead, REM bursts onto the sleep scene before it has been invited. Nearly three out of four narcoleptics begin their sleep cycles with a REM phase, unlike normal people, whose first REM period may not come for an hour or more after onset of sleep. The overall percentage of REM sleep is the same, but the periods are fragmented. Researchers are investigating the possible role in triggering narcoleptic attacks played by acetylcholine, the neurotransmitter thought to be involved with instigating the REM phase. One other clue to the cause may be the fact that narcoleptics show increased blood flow in the brain, especially through the brain stem, where REM sleep is regulated. (Other aspects of sleep architecture are also affected by narcolepsy: those with the disorder fall asleep much more quickly when they go to bed—usually within five minutes or less, compared with fifteen to thirty minutes for normal individuals.)

Abnormal REM sleep may account to one extent or another for most of the classic symptoms of narcolepsy. For example, experiencing dream-filled REM sleep immediately after dropping off may be perceived and reported by the sleeper as a hallucination.

Also, as we have seen, a mechanism exists to suppress muscle activity and prevent us from acting out our REM dreams. When a narcoleptic experiences a sudden burst of REM sleep, this muscle suppressant may suddenly be activated, which in turn may trigger cataplexy or sleep paralysis.

Identifying Narcolepsy

Diagnosis of narcolepsy is sometimes slow to occur. Until recently the average interval between first appearance of symptoms and diagnosis was as long as thirteen years. During that time inappropriate therapy, such as psychotherapy, may have been attempted, usually to no avail since such an approach obviously does not address the cause of the problem. Sometimes the symptoms of narcolepsy are mistaken for withdrawal from society, lack of motivation, poor or negative attitude, hostility, or just plain laziness. Hallucinations are occasionally misinterpreted as stemming from a psychological disorder or, in some cases, use of drugs. Depression is a factor for one out of three narcoleptics, primarily because of the disruption in their lives and the feeling that they are denied the right to enjoy many of life's experiences.

Diagnosis is made more difficult by the wide range of severity of the disorder. As I noted earlier, some victims do not exhibit cataplexy, the one telltale sign that the disease is present. What's more, patients may occasionally experience a temporary or partial remission in their condition. However, if I suspect that narcolepsy is present, I may refer the patient for a multiple sleep latency test, which records sleep patterns during several daytime naps over the course of a few hours. Such a test is easy, convenient, inexpensive, and very informative. As we have seen, sleep patterns, especially the presence of the REM phase immediately after onset of sleep, can help confirm the diagnosis.

Management of Narcolepsy

There are several therapeutic options that can help relieve the symptoms of narcolepsy. Such stimulant drugs as methylphenidate (brand name Ritalin) or pemoline (Cylert) may help relieve feelings of drowsiness. Tricyclic antidepressants (such as protriptyline and imipramine) can alleviate cataplexy. It may be months, however, before the positive effects of drug therapy are fully experienced. Sometimes, unlike epileptic seizures, narcoleptic attacks can be arrested by stimulating the victim through talking or gentle shaking. In many cases maintaining a regular sleep-wake schedule and arranging periodic naps can help minimize the number of daytime attacks. Supportive counseling can work wonders in helping narcoleptics adjust to their situation, especially if situational depression is present. However, as I mentioned, many forms of psychotherapy, such as drug management for depression, are obviously inappropriate, since they do not address the cause of narcolepsy.

OTHER TYPES OF DOES

If you experience a period of excessive sleepiness, you may find that it, like other sleep disorders, is a response to a transient life situation, such as conflict, loss, grief, or stress. If so, your problem will usually resolve itself within a short time. The need for additional sleep may even be therapeutic to some extent, serving to gently remove you from conscious awareness of your problem and perhaps allowing you the opportunity for further restorative sleep. However, if you find that the sleepiness persists for longer than two or three weeks, or if it begins to interfere with your daytime functioning, you should seek the advice of a physician.

If no evidence of sleep apnea or narcolepsy can be found, then some other cause for excessive daytime sleepiness must be identified. Although seen relatively infrequently, any of the following types of DOES may be the source of difficulty in staying awake and functioning fully during the day.

Psychiatric DOES

Sometimes excessive sleepiness can mask the presence of depression, especially if the depression is of the type known as bipolar or manic-depressive illness (where periods of euphoria or mania are followed by depressed periods). As we have seen, however, the more common type of depression, classified as unipolar, usually results in a different sleep problem, that of early-morning insomnia.

Besides depression, there are other, far less common, psychiatric conditions that may include excessive daytime sleepiness as a symptom. Generally these are the dissociative disorders in which the victim loses touch with reality through amnesia or some other cause. An example is the fugue state, in which victims suddenly lose all recollection of past or current life, usually wandering off to begin a totally new existence with a new identity in a new location, completely unaware that anything has changed. After a few days or weeks these individuals will suddenly "come to," returning to their prior identity, unable to remember how they got where they are. Needless to say, such conditions, while fortunately rare, can be extremely distressing. Hypersomnia is also present in many cases of schizophrenia and in borderline personality disorders.

Pathophysiological DOES—learned behavior in which the pattern of daytime sleepiness is reinforced by habit—is much less common than the bad sleep habits that may be associated with insomnia. For short intervals of time some people may take to their beds as a minor depressive response to an event, or to escape the pressures of living. They may thus come to depend on such escape on a regular basis, conditioning themselves to expect sleepiness to occur with a certain frequency. Such a pattern seldom extends over the long term, although in some cases it can develop into a persistent complaint of chronic weariness, excessive sleep, and daytime napping. Thorough clinical examination, including a visit to a sleep lab, will usually reveal no objective findings to suggest a cause for the hypersomnia. Supportive counseling to address the initial reason for sleepiness and to change the pattern of behavior is called for.

Drugs and Alcohol

Much more frequently substance abuse—particularly abuse of alcohol—is the root of a hypersomnia complaint not caused by apnea or narcolepsy. Stimulant drugs, including amphetamines and appetite suppressants, can lead to dependence. When tolerance builds up to a certain point, or if the user withdraws from the substance, the consequences may include sleepiness, sleep attacks, impaired arousal, or extended sleep at night. Other drugs that have hypersomnia as a frequent side effect include long-acting benzodiazepines, some oral contraceptives, muscle relaxants, antihistamines, and tricyclic and reserpine antidepressants. Heroin affects the central nervous system; addicts are notorious for their constant tendency to nod off during the day.

In evaluating patients who complain of hypersomnia, I will sometimes have to probe deeply to uncover use of some of these substances. If you suffer from excessive sleepiness, take a long, careful look at your habits to see if the cause might be chemical in origin. If so, and if you subsequently find you are unable to change your behavior through your own efforts, a medical professional can help you take advantage of the many psychological and supportive therapies that have proved helpful to millions of people. I'll describe these in greater detail in Chapter 10.

Nocturnal Myoclonus

As we saw earlier, nighttime leg-twitching can disrupt sleep. Sometimes, though, victims are not sufficiently aroused to classify the problem as one of insomnia—the inability to sleep. In those cases the consequence of myoclonus takes the form of excessive daytime sleepiness. According to one study, about 3.5 percent of patients had hypersomnia attributable to myoclonus and restless legs syndrome. By observing your sleep over the course of a night, a sleep lab can make a concrete determination as to whether leg jerks are contributing to your hypersomnia. Some researchers also feel that the same neurological abnormality that causes myoclonus may also contribute directly, in some way, to feelings of daytime sleepiness.

"Sleep Drunkenness"

I like to describe this condition as a "severe case of Monday morning, every day of the week." Victims, mostly male, undergo a prolonged time of transition between sleeping and wakefulness. In some cases their feelings of sleepiness can last until noon or later. During that interval their movements may be clumsy or uncoordinated, their ability to make decisions is reduced, and the few judgments they do make are cloudy or inappropriate. Obviously such a pattern can impair one's ability to function. I recently counseled a patient who was extremely distraught because she was fired from her job as a secretary after her boss publicly accused her of drinking on the job. A lifelong teetotaler and devoutly religious person, she had to cope with extreme feelings of shame, anger, and depression. Psychological and supportive counseling were called for; another strategy that proved helpful, she reported, was finding a split-shift job that allowed her to begin work at one in the afternoon. Unfortunately, her condition of delayed morning arousal still persists.

While there is insufficient research on this syndrome to understand it thoroughly, it appears to arise from a malfunction in the arousal mechanism of the brain, and it may be an inherited trait. The urine of a sleep-drunk patient often shows low levels of homovanillic acid, a by-product of dopamine, which is a neurotransmitter involved in the arousal process. Experts interpret this finding to mean that victims of sleep drunkenness have reduced amounts of this crucial chemical. The problem is made worse if the victim is forced to awaken during Stage 3 or 4 of the sleep cycle. Sleep deprivation, physical fatigue, or use of some drugs can also compound the problem. Some victims find that abstaining from stimulants, including coffee, can make it easier to stir in the morning.

Sleep Paralysis

As we have seen, narcoleptics occasionally experience muscle paralysis associated with the onset or termination of sleep. The same problem can afflict nonnarcoleptic people as well. Patients lie unable to move any muscles, except those around the eyes. In some cases the victim suffers formication—the frightening sense that bugs are crawling over the body—or other hallucinations. Sleep paralysis, which is inherited through the mother, may be a dysfunction of the REM mechanism responsible for inhibiting muscle movement during dreams. There may also be a dietary basis for the problem in hypokalemic individuals—those with low or depleted levels of potassium, an electrolyte necessary for muscle function.

If you suffer from an attack of sleep paralysis, concentrate on moving your eyes as vigorously as you can. Blink, if possible. Then try moving individual muscles in your face, slowly and systematically working your way down your body. Such activity has been shown to terminate the paralysis.

Kleine-Levin Syndrome

This rare cause of hypersomnia usually affects males, most often between the ages of ten and twenty-one. Victims experience bouts of extreme daytime sleepiness coupled with unusual eating patterns. The fact that victims alternate between periods of enormous appetite and near starvation leads some authorities to suspect that the cause of the syndrome lies in a malfunctioning appetite control center in the brain. Other behavior helps differentiate this syndrome: irritability, confusion, incoherent speech, delusions, social isolation, shyness, and apathy. Victims may demonstrate exceptionally aggressive or inappropriate sexual activity, such as exhibitionism. Metabolic disturbances can be detected through urinalysis. Victims experience earlier and shorter REM periods and less deep NREM sleep. After a period of time the condition enters a stage of remission that can last months or even years. Sleep during this time is normal. Diagnosis of this unusual condition is tricky, since some of these symptoms may appear to be just part of the transition from prepubescence to young adulthood. Indeed, there may be some connection to the rampaging hormonal activity of this stage of life. Treatment with lithium carbonate may prevent (but not eliminate) attacks; the condition usually resolves itself spontaneously before the age of forty.

The Menstrual Cycle and Pregnancy

At certain times in the hormonal cycle of a woman, especially an adolescent, she may feel particularly drowsy or lethargic. In rare and extreme cases the cycle can produce bizarre behavior, including voracious appetite or unusual sexual activity, similar to that seen in men with Kleine-Levin syndrome. After menopause, another period of hormonal turbulence, deep sleep declines dramatically, which may lead to feelings of daytime somnolence.

Also, excessive sleepiness may be an early sign of pregnancy. Expectant mothers almost always extend their total daily sleep, usually by as much as two hours, throughout their pregnancies. As most mothers know, the effects of hormonal disruption can last for months after the baby is born. The desire to sleep persists, but the opportunity—what with nighttime feedings, diaper changes, and other changes in lifestyle—is no longer there. One of my patients jokingly told me she had designed the perfect cure for parental hypersomnia: send the kid to college. This therapeutic approach has drawbacks, she admitted: it's expensive, and it usually takes eighteen years before you can actually begin the treatment.

"Long Sleeper" Syndrome

People who fit this category simply sleep longer than average compared to others in their age group—usually for nine to fourteen hours. They demonstrate a normal sleep cycle and seem to have no physiological problem. Nor do they usually complain about excessive sleepiness; any problem arising from their condition is connected to fears that they may be psychologically or medically abnormal. The demands placed on them by work load or social activities, however, may prevent them from obtaining the amount of sleep they need in order to feel adequately rested.

The Pickwickian Syndrome

This is so called because of a character in Charles Dickens's *The Pickwick Papers.* Joe—described as a "natural curiosity"— is an overweight boy who is able to sleep as he runs errands or waits on his master. The Pickwickian syndrome applies to obese people who are shallow breathers. These individuals are victims of a vicious circle: they tend to retain carbon dioxide in their blood, and this retention causes a decrease in the ability of CO_2 to act as a stimulant to the respiratory drive. Reduced central functioning in turn means that less oxygen enters the bloodstream. The end result is hypersomnolence. Erythrocytosis (abnormal red blood cell mass) is another common finding among Pickwickians. Progesterone and related compounds are sometimes successful in increasing ventilation.

Other Forms of DOES

Hypersomnia is often reported as a symptom of a number of other disorders. Space doesn't permit a detailed discussion of each one, but the following conditions should be considered if no other cause of sleepiness can be found.

* Central nervous system (CNS) disorders: Hypothyroidism is the most likely cause; other possibilities include encephalitis, tumor, increased intracranial pressure, neurosyphilis, hydrocephalus (progressive accumulation of fluid within the skull), lesions, hemorrhage, trauma or other brain injury. CNS hypersomnia seems to be related to the presence of high levels of a product of the neurotransmitter serotonin. Drugs that inhibit serotonin production thus have demonstrated some effectiveness against excessive daytime sleepiness.
* Endocrine and metabolic disorders such as hypoglycemia and diabetes
* Nutritional deficiencies, including skipping breakfast
* Other medical conditions: Uremia, anemia, degenerative brain disease caused by dysfunctions in the liver, hematoma (pooling of blood), postsurgical complications, pain, a change in dose or timing of drug regimens
* Social conditions such as boredom, isolation, or confinement

Idiopathic Hypersomnia

"Idiopathic" comes from a Latin word that, in rough translation, means "we don't know what causes it." As an example of this poorly defined disorder, let me cite the incident of a patient whose nightly ritual after dinner was to load the dishwasher and take out the garbage. One night before retiring, however, she went to unload the dishwasher—and found the sealed plastic bag of garbage sitting in it, all freshly washed, rinsed, and dried. She found the dinner dishes, of course, in the garbage can. To this day we don't know what caused her problem.

Also called non-REM narcolepsy, idiopathic hypersomnia can make patients feel constantly sleepy without overwhelming them with sleep attacks or cataplexy. Sufferers usually sleep well at night, although their sleep may be prolonged and they may have difficulty rousing. If they take naps, as they often do, the naps are long and unrefreshing. Clinical tests reveal that these patients fall asleep relatively quickly, but REM sleep is not usually present during naps as it is in narcolepsy. In some cases treatment with CNS stimulants or methysergide (Sansert) may help.

Poor Sleep Hygiene

As we have seen, bad habits such as frequent naps, irregular sleeping and waking schedules, or too much time in bed can exacerbate daytime sleepiness. Such behavior can disrupt circadian rhythms—for example, body temperature and endocrine function—which then become entrained to different periodic cycles and lose their normal, predictable nature. A closer look at disturbed rhythms follows.

DISORDERS OF THE SLEEP-WAKE SCHEDULE (DSWS)

While strictly speaking this category is diagnostically different from DOES, a discussion is appropriate at this point because one of the chief symptoms of DSWS is sleepiness during the day.

Generally all DSWS problems involve some kind of misalignment between the normal twenty-four-hour organization of the sleep-wake schedule and the patient's internal circadian rhythm. In other words, through some dysfunction or other, a person's internal system may persistently operate on a cycle with a period significantly greater or less than the twenty-four hours mandated by the earth's daily rotation. Most of our circadian rhythms operate on a cycle that lasts roughly twenty-five hours. Patients with DSWS, however, experience abnormal rhythms. In these people, the abnormal period may be as few as twenty hours or as many as thirty to forty. Obviously, such an intrinsically out-of-whack schedule can wreak havoc for an individual struggling to maintain a normal life within a society based on a twenty-four-hour clock.

Although chronobiology is a relatively new branch of the relatively young science of sleep research, experts, with their typical zeal for classification and categorization, have already delineated a number of different types of DSWS. The most commonly seen varieties of DSWS—jet lag and the negative effects of shift work—have already been discussed in some detail. At this point, then, let me simply reiterate that travelers to new time zones (especially those who are eastbound) or people who work at odd hours are prone to disruptions in a number of circadian rhythms, including adrenaline, heart rate, body temperature, and alertness, which result in feelings of disorientation and malaise. As we have seen, endogenous sleep-wake cycles are also affected. A number of time-management, dietary, and drug strategies can help modify the effects of these life-disrupting conditions.

Delayed Sleep Phase Syndrome

All of us at times stay up later than we want to or later than we should—cramming for tests, completing projects for work, or enjoying a late-night social event. Usually we have no trouble readjusting to our normal schedule. If our sleep cycle is biologically delayed, however, we may find it virtually impossible to go to sleep at a "normal" or reasonable time. More often seen in young adults, delayed sleep phase syndrome (or, if you'll permit me yet another acronym, DSPS) often causes its victims to go to bed before they're really ready to sleep, in a futile effort to operate on a regular schedule. Once in bed, they are unable to drop off for an extended time—perhaps an hour or more. They usually sleep normally once sleep has come, but naturally they find it very difficult to rise and function in the morning. Given a choice, these patients would usually sleep from about three in the morning to about noon the following day. Because they often must be at work by eight or nine o'clock, however, they leave their beds too soon, depriving themselves of necessary rest. This form of sleep deprivation may have other effects which make the actual diagnosis of delayed sleep phase more difficult. One clue, however, is that DSPS sufferers may look forward to weekends because, as one patient put it, "I can get up at the crack of noon."

DSPS is estimated to affect some 7 to 10 percent of insomniacs. Physicians must be careful to distinguish it from difficulty initiating sleep, a different problem whose therapy—hypnotic drugs—is inappropriate in treating DSPS victims. One strategy that does seem to work is called chronotherapy. In this process patients are told to delay their bedtimes significantly—by three hours or so per night over a five- or six-day period. Thus, the first night, the patient might retire at midnight; the next night, at 3:00 A.M., and so on. Eventually, patients "catch up" with their cycles, resetting their internal clocks so that they are able to retire, and fall asleep, on a more normal schedule. One late night, however, can disrupt the pattern and result in recurrence of the disorder.

Prolonged Sleep-Wake Cycles

Victims of this form of sleep disruption may experience a circadian sleep cycle lasting as long as thirty-five to forty hours—an exaggerated form of delayed sleep phase syndrome in which victims may feel like sleeping only once every day and a half or so. But as is not the case with DSPS, whose pattern remains relatively fixed over time, patients with prolonged cycles experience a pattern of incremental delays in sleep-wake times. In other words, sleep may befall the patient at noon on one day, at 6:00 P.M. the next, and at midnight the day after that. The chief complaint of these patients is difficulty falling asleep at a normal time, coupled with inability to remain awake during the day. Interestingly, this pattern is often found in blind individuals, who lack access to light—which, as we have seen, is the most common time cue for setting the circadian clock. Schizophrenic patients, isolated from normal social time clues, may also exhibit prolonged cycles.

Advanced Sleep Phase Syndrome (ASPS)

As its name suggests, ASPS is the flip side of delayed sleep; it is more common among the middle-aged. Victims of ASPS may fall asleep as early as 8:00 or 9:00 P.M. and awaken in the early hours of the morning, usually after a normal night's sleep. They begin to feel fatigued by late afternoon—the equivalent of about ten o'clock at night for most of us—and are unable to stay awake during the evening or to sleep until daybreak. As you can see, ASPS is a different problem from the early-morning insomnia described earlier, in which the patient may retire at midnight and still rise at four in the morning.

One potentially effective treatment is the mirror image of chronotherapy. The patient is asked to systematically restrict the amount of sleep each night in order to lengthen the period of wakefulness before the next sleep period. Thus, the first night, the patient may retire at 8:30 instead of 8:00; the second night, bedtime is 9:00; and so on. This gradual approach helps some ASPS patients to eventually adapt to a later sleep schedule, one more amenable to their lifestyle and that of their family and friends.

Irregular Sleep Phase Syndrome

This pattern describes patients whose sleep cycles fit none of the unusual, although regular and predictable, patterns described above. These patients experience random, wildly fluctuating sleep behavior, marked by excessive periods in bed at different hours every day, coupled with frequent daytime naps. Unlike victims of the other syndromes, they do not sleep long enough at night, although over a period of twenty-four hours they may obtain normal rest (i.e., eight hours' worth). Therapy may take a variety of forms, including supportive counseling, behavioral counseling, or drugs, in an effort to reset and restrain the circadian pattern.

As with any sleep disorder, however, the specific approach taken toward its management must of course be determined by the results of careful and thorough physical, medical, and psychiatric examination. In addition, the findings derived from analysis by a sleep laboratory can be invaluable—if not crucial—in understanding the true nature of the problem and outlining a course of effective therapy.

7

Parasomnias: From Sleepwalking to Sleeptalking

Up to now the sleep disorders we have examined are those involving disruptions in the physiological process of falling asleep or maintaining sleep and those involving the daytime consequences of disturbed sleep. At this point let's turn our attention to phenomena that are not directly related to malfunctions of the sleep process itself but can interfere with, or are exacerbated by, sleep. Such disorders, some of which affect children almost exclusively, are given the name "parasomnias," a word that translates roughly as "events associated with sleep." Parasomnias account for nearly one out of ten diagnoses of sleep disorders.

Parasomnias are disorders involving unwanted or abnormal events, including sleepwalking, bed-wetting, and behaviors such as teeth grinding or head banging. (While nightmares and the panic disorder known as night terrors are also forms of parasomnia, they will be covered in Chapter 12 in order to place them in the larger context of dreams and dream states.) A patient with a parasomnia will usually complain about the problem itself— bed-wetting, for example—rather than about the disturbed sleep the problem is causing.

Generally speaking, the cluster of parasomnia disorders tends to occur at the threshold between wakefulness and sleep, or during deep sleep—Stages 3 and 4 of the sleep cycle. And, because the longest periods of deep sleep occur in the first part of the cycle, most parasomnia events tend to take place early in the night, usually about an hour after the onset of sleep. I use the term "cluster" because often more than one form of the disorder afflicts the same person. For example, the same problem that is manifested as sleepwalking may also be the underlying cause of bed-wetting.

As I mentioned, children and early adolescents are the usual victims of parasomnias. The younger your child, the more likely the occurrence: about 20 percent of two-year-olds wake at night due to one of these sleep disturbances. The rate declines slightly in children aged three and four but persists at a rate of about 10 percent in children of four and a half. Most of these conditions vanish by later adolescence. In severe cases, however, they can cause a number of problems if left untreated. Obviously, the sufferer gets less sleep than is needed—especially dangerous during these crucial developmental years. What's more, a sleepy child is often unfairly branded as lazy, disobedient, retarded, or emotionally disturbed. Naturally, such a child is at risk of developing poor morale, low self-esteem, and a negative or hopeless attitude. Academic performance may begin to suffer; when that happens, the child may be classified as learning disabled or as an underachiever—a stigma that can affect the educational process for years and prevent children from realizing their full potential.

Parasomnias, as a rule, are age-related, occurring with fairly predictable frequency at certain stages of development. For infants the cause of sleep disturbance is most likely to be either colic, persistent crying, or the habitual expectation of night feeding. In children between the ages of one and three, the most common problems are difficulty falling asleep or waking up; resisting sleep due to fear of separation; loss of bladder control; thumb sucking; and rocking. Between the ages of four and six, children are more prone to classic parasomnias such as head banging, rocking, night terrors, sleepwalking, and bed-wetting. Six- to twelve-year-olds are more subject to stress, anxiety, and bad dreams. Adolescents demonstrate a higher incidence of daytime sleepiness and extended nocturnal sleep.

Possible Causes of Parasomnias

If your child suffers from a parasomnia disorder, you the parent may bear part of the responsibility: to a significant extent, parasomnias are an inherited trait. In one study, for example, nearly four out of five adults who walked in their sleep reported that other members of their families had similar problems.

Some authorities feel that parents may be responsible in other ways as well. As evidence they point to the bedtime techniques used by parents in the "developed" world and compare them with those of other cultures. For example, it is considered normal by many cultures to allow the child to sleep in the parents' bed, not only for the child's peace of mind but to facilitate breast-feeding as well. In such cases children may feel more secure and thus sleep more soundly; nighttime wakings occur less often, are more easily dealt with, and disturb other family members to a lesser extent.

Some well-meaning parents may also inadvertently contribute to the problem by rushing in to comfort or feed children every time they stir. In doing so, they may be encouraging them to awaken regularly and unnecessarily. As we have seen, however, everyone experiences brief periods of wakefulness as a response to troubling events or temporary situations. What's more, it is natural to awaken several times at night, usually at the end of a complete sleep cycle. Also, many parents rock children in a chair or allow them to fall asleep in the parents' bed, then move them to their own crib. A child who falls asleep in one place and wakes up in another may feel confused or frightened and may thus cry out in hopes of having the previous sleep situation restored. Parents nowadays are counseled to show appropriate concern for the child's wakefulness without reinforcing temporary or natural waking behavior and turning it into a learned habit.

In addition to heredity and habit, causes of parasomnia may involve such factors as sleep hygiene, medical disorders, central nervous system abnormalities, or lifestyle patterns such as diet or daytime activity level. If I suspect that your problem or your child's is a parasomnia disorder, I will try to obtain a thorough family, social, and developmental history and a detailed assess-

ment of personality, in addition to the medical history, in order
to paint as complete a picture of the problem as possible. Doing
so will help rule out such conditions as narcolepsy or a sleep-
related breathing disorder. It may also reveal whether the cause
of the nighttime arousal is relatively apparent, such as noisy
neighbors or insufficient nutrition, or is more deeply rooted,
stemming from family stress or from a chemical imbalance in
the brain.

Depending on the cause and nature of the problem, there are
a number of therapies and management techniques that can
help minimize or eliminate the consequences of the various parasomnias. Let's look now at these disorders and what can be done
about them.

SLEEPWALKING

Perhaps the strangest of all sleep disorders is sleepwalking,
more technically known as somnambulism. Many of us can recall incidents where we, or our relatives, were discovered wandering about the house, seemingly wide awake but behaving in
bizarre, funny, or sometimes dangerous ways. Come morning,
sleepwalkers are completely unaware of their nocturnal peram-
bulations and frequently wince as others recount the tales of
their outrageous activities.

Sleepwalking episodes are probably directly related to deep
sleep. The most striking symptom of the condition, of course, is
what researchers call intense autonomic activation—or, in layman's terms, unconscious movement. Sleepwalking activity may
last anywhere from five minutes to half an hour but usually less
than ten minutes. Walkers wear blank expressions (and sometimes not much else). They seem indifferent to the environment,
for example, ignoring freezing cold and traipsing barefoot in the
snow. Physically awake but mentally asleep, they demonstrate
only a minimal level of awareness and reactivity but do exhibit
some skill in maneuvering around objects. They know they are
walking down steps, for example, and can open doors or use tools
appropriately. By and large, however, their activity is purpose-
less and clumsy; they are unable to play the piano, for instance,

or to prepare a meal. Somnambulists' eyes are open, but they don't see. A sleepwalker may talk, more or less coherently.

As I indicated, a genetic factor is one primary reason why some people sleepwalk and others don't. In a study of military personnel, 56 percent of the sailors who sleepwalked reported having relatives with the same tendency; by contrast, not one of sixty sailors who stayed anchored to their berths had sleepwalking relatives. Medical literature records the case of a patient who was descended from a long line of somnambulists. During one family gathering at Christmastime he awakened to find himself surrounded by sleeping aunts and uncles, who had all gathered in the dining room for an impromptu nocturnal reunion.

About 15 percent of children sleepwalk at least once in their lives, and between 3 and 6 percent do so more often. By way of comparison, only about 2 to 5 percent of adults experience one or more sleepwalking adventures; less than 1 percent do so with any frequency. Interestingly, children who are known sleepwalkers and who have reached the deep sleep stage and are lifted to a standing position are likely to begin moving about. (*Please* take my word and don't experiment with this; I don't want to be accused of being responsible for encouraging the launching of an entire armada of wandering youngsters.)

The sleepwalking behavior that begins in childhood frequently and almost inevitably ends by late adolescence. Boys are somewhat more likely to sleepwalk than girls, and the pattern of walking will also persist longer among males. The fact that sleepwalking behavior beginning in adulthood is extremely rare suggests that it is tied to some aspect of the maturing process. Indeed, EEG tracings of children who sleepwalk reveal a distinctive pattern of sudden, rhythmic, high-voltage slow-wave activity, a pattern researchers call the immaturity factor.

Very rarely there may be an organic element as well: the presence of fever or a brain tumor might trigger sleepwalking activity. Adult sleepwalking is more likely to involve some psychological factor, such as stress, emotional tension, or a significant life event like the death of a loved one. Interestingly, many sleepwalkers report noticing a strange "electrical" feeling right before they go to sleep, a feeling which forewarns them that they will probably sleepwalk that night. The use of lithium, often prescribed for the management of manic-depressive disorders, or high doses of neuroleptic drugs and the benzodiazepine triazolam or other sleeping medications have been associated with incidents of sleepwalking. People who have been deprived of sleep are also potential victims.

Obviously, a diagnosis of sleepwalking is not terribly difficult, although it usually depends on anecdotal evidence from concerned parents or relatives. In assessing your condition, I will try to determine the age at which your problem began and whether there may have been some kind of stressful event at about the same time. Other questions will focus on how often you walk and for how long, and whether any daytime behavior patterns exist that may provide further clues. Basically my goal is simply to eliminate the possible presence of other types of disorders—those caused by fever, for example, or such extreme and rare psychiatric problems as amnesia, multiple personalities, or fugue states in which victims temporarily take up entirely new lives. I may order neurological tests to rule out a diagnosis of epilepsy; psychological evaluation may also help uncover a reason for the behavior.

Often victims of sleepwalking are also prey to episodes of night terrors, a disorder characterized by extreme panic and the physical reactions that accompany it, such as increased heartbeat or sweating. In fact, it is thought that sleepwalking is a milder form of the same pathophysiology that generates night terrors. As we'll see in Chapter 12, night terrors tend to occur during the same stage of sleep as somnambulism, usually during the first hours after retiring.

Management of Sleepwalking

My approach to managing sleepwalking is usually one of benign neglect. Children almost always outgrow the problem between the ages of seven and fourteen, with no permanent psychological damage, while virtually any kind of treatment may be worse than the condition itself. Drugs are usually of little value and may produce unwanted side effects. Psychological counseling or behavior modification is a two-edged sword; such an approach may work in some children, while in others it may produce undue anxiety. Maintaining a regular sleep schedule helps.

Time and patience, however, are the best remedies. Some form of family counseling may also help reassure the parents that the child is not suffering from any serious disorder.

In adult sleepwalkers there may be an element of emotional disturbance which does need to be addressed. If so, careful psychiatric evaluation is needed to determine which approach has the greatest chance of success. Benzodiazepine drugs such as diazepam and flurazepam may help, primarily due to the fact that they suppress Stages 3 and 4 sleep. Evidence of any benefit from a drug called imipramine, used in the treatment of endogenous depression and childhood bed-wetting, is still inconclusive. It's also possible that hypnotism, conducted by a qualified professional, may produce some benefits, although many investigators feel it will not work.

Sleepwalking Tips

The following are some practical steps you can take if you are concerned about a sleepwalker in your family.

* Accidents can happen, so it's advisable to lock all windows and doors.
* If possible, have the sleepwalker sleep on the first floor.
* Hide the keys to the car, and don't tell the walker where they are.
* Block passageways, especially near stairs.

Opinions vary as to whether you should wake a sleepwalker. As a rule, there's no need to do so; as you can imagine, being awakened suddenly and finding yourself in strange surroundings can be frightening or upsetting. If you can, simply guide the walker back to bed, speaking in reassuring tones. The exception, of course, is if danger is imminent. In that case call the walker's name several times in a firm tone until your voice penetrates his or her consciousness. Give reassurance that everything is fine, and help the walker return to bed.

Finally, before leaving the subject of sleepwalking, let me share with you two of my favorite anecdotes from the annals of sleepwalking. The first concerns a baronet who would go to sleep every night wearing a bed shirt but awaken to find himself completely naked. Hundreds of shirts thus disappeared until the man posted a friend to try to catch the thief. It turned out that every night, as the clock struck one, the baronet had risen, wandered into the yard, and, using a pitchfork, buried his nightshirt in a dunghill before returning, au naturel, to his bed.

The second story involves a British woman, staying in one of the stately homes of England, who recalled the night she awakened and heard the distinct—and terrifying—sounds of a man moving about the room. Every so often she felt him touch the bed. Eventually, unable to bear the tension, she fainted. On awakening the next morning, she discovered that the butler had walked in his sleep and had laid out formal place settings for fourteen people—using her bed as the table.

BED-WETTING

Bed-wetting (also called enuresis) is defined as nighttime urination that occurs after the age at which bladder control should have been achieved—usually, between three and four. However, due to differences in children, I consider bed-wetting to be abnormal only in children of five or older. About 10 percent of children between the ages of three and ten are enuretic; the figure drops to around 3 percent in twelve-year-olds. It's difficult to determine the incidence in adults, since many will not admit to the problem, but estimates range from 1 to 3 percent. Boys are more likely to suffer from enuresis, and for longer periods of time.

Children's central nervous systems are not yet fully developed; consequently, they are more prone to nighttime disturbances stemming from their environment as well as from some fluctuation in their physiological functioning. Bed-wetting usually occurs during such a disturbance, when the child experiences a brief, partial awakening. Like other forms of parasomnia, enuresis is related to the deep stage of sleep; two out of three incidents occur in the first third of the night. Contrary to popular belief, bed-wetting is for the most part unconnected to dreams or the REM stage.

Urologists describe two basic categories of bed-wetting. Primary (or persistent) enuresis, the most common, is considered to be present if the child is unable to stop bed-wetting for more than a month—in other words, if the child has never really learned how to stay dry. Secondary (acquired or "regressed") enuresis appears after a dry period lasting months or even years; in this case, the child has regressed in behavior, usually due to some psychological factor.

Primary enuresis, which is pretty common up to the age of five, may be simply the result of large fluid intake, coupled with the inability to rouse oneself completely to make the trip to the bathroom. There may be a family history of the problem. One major contributing factor may be a small bladder, which is incapable of holding enough urine to avoid the need to urinate before sleep has ended. In more serious cases, however, bed-wetting may be a symptom of diabetes, nocturnal epilepsy, retardation, or some form of neurologic disorder.

Secondary enuresis, on the other hand, usually arises from some kind of emotional trauma—the birth of a sibling, for example, or the stress of the parents' divorce. Such behavior may be little more than a regressive cry for help or attention. However, a physical cause may need to be ruled out, since such medical problems as pinworms, infection, sickle-cell anemia, or urinary tract disorders can cause the sudden onset of bed-wetting behavior. Enuresis is also a possible consequence of obstructive sleep apnea.

As with other parasomnias, your family and medical histories are crucial pieces of evidence in the diagnosis of enuresis. Of particular relevance is the age of onset and the interval between bed-wetting episodes. Physical examination should include an observation of the patient's urine stream, which may reveal clues about the internal functioning of the urinary system. Urinalysis will suggest whether any metabolic malfunction has occurred. I would also be sure to rule out any infection or renal disease that may be the cause of the problem. There are a few simple tests I might use to assess bladder capacity.

Another particularly vital clue might emerge from my conversation with you concerning your attitudes toward your child's toilet teaching. Are you particularly adamant that your child perform to a certain high level of expectation? Or are you blasé to the point of indifference about your child's toilet habits, failing to reinforce certain basic toilet teaching behavior? Either way, your children's voiding performance may be directly related to the signals you are giving about what is expected of them. If your child is a problem bed-wetter, I suggest you first examine your own attitudes about toilet teaching to see if you may be applying undue or premature pressure. A conversation with your family physician, a urologist, or a psychologist may help correct bad or harmful habits.

If bed-wetting persists into adolescence, a psychological evaluation is necessary to determine the possible cause; nocturnal incontinence is a factor in about 3.6 percent of cases of psychosis. In middle-aged or elderly patients, I would also order neurological tests in order to rule out certain conditions, including epilepsy and other seizure disorders, which may be robbing them of bladder control. I would also look for signs of excessive daytime sleepiness, since one consequence of a DOES complaint may be the inability to rouse oneself sufficiently during the night.

Management of Bed-wetting

Appropriate treatment of bed-wetting depends, of course, on the specific cause of the problem. In children perhaps the most important thing you can do is avoid overreacting to the situation. Children who wet the bed are not necessarily psychologically disturbed. Just the opposite: they are more likely to suffer psychological damage as a *result* of bed-wetting, due to the shame and embarrassment they experience among their family and friends. Your ability to deal patiently and rationally with the problem may be greatly enhanced by a simple tip: try double-layering the bed with regular and rubber sheets (one rubber sheet, followed by a regular sheet, followed by a rubber sheet, and topped off with a regular sheet). That way if bed-wetting occurs, you can quickly remove the top two sheets, return to sleep, and still feel confident that if the bed-wetting happens again you won't have to confront a urine-soaked mattress. Your patience and understanding are the essential ingredients of any therapeutic approach.

Some management strategy is usually called for, however. The rate of spontaneous cure of bed-wetting is only about 15 percent per year in children over the age of six. The rest need some kind of thoughtful intervention in order to help remedy the situation.

As I often tell the concerned parents who seek my advice, correcting the unwanted behavior is only part of the goal. The other, and perhaps more critical, element is to demonstrate your awareness of, and sensitivity to, the needs of your children while they are awake.

Simply educating and reassuring both you and your bed-wetting child can work wonders. When parents are counseled to avoid harsh and punitive reactions that can create anxiety, guilt, or anger and may actually worsen the problem, they are then better able to try more productive strategies. Psychotherapeutic management is especially appropriate in cases of secondary enuresis, as it may reveal some stressful event in the child's life that has caused bed-wetting behavior to develop.

Motivational counseling works to effect a cure in about one out of four bed-wetters. In this approach, children are encouraged to experience directly the consequences of their actions. If they are physically able, for example, they are asked to dress themselves in fresh pajamas and change their own wet bedsheets. Giving the child special rewards for staying dry—using a calendar marked with gold stars or serving favorite breakfast foods—may work.

Behavioral techniques often prove effective. The child may be given bladder-stretching exercises, thus learning to become more aware of bodily signals. The technique of drinking large amounts of fluid and then refraining from urination for as long as possible helps improve functional bladder capacity, enabling the child to go for longer periods between voidings. Also, stream interruption exercises—stopping and starting the flow of urine— serve to improve the tone of the muscles that control the urinary sphincter and help make the child aware of the techniques necessary to control the voiding process. Studies show that stream interruption exercises alone can produce remission of enuresis in as many as 35 percent of cases. The process of visual sequencing—training the child to mentally envision and rehearse the process of waking and going to the toilet—can also help. Some experts suggest keeping a bedpan nearby to make voiding easier. Even reducing the amount of spicy or salty foods in the diet produces some results.

A number of bed-wetting alarm systems are available from such retailers as Sears. Some of these are connected to the mattress; others fit inside the underpants, with the alarm worn on the wrist. Battery-operated and triggered by the first signs of urination, buzzers and lights rouse the child, who is trained to stop the flow and make the pilgrimage to the bathroom. Considered by some to be the most effective management option available, such devices cost between $50 and $70 and post a success rate of about 70 percent. At least one study has demonstrated that alarms are more effective than therapy with imipramine (see below). A cheaper and somewhat less technical approach is to have the parents note the time at which bed-wetting episodes seem to occur, and set an alarm clock to go off a few minutes before that time. The idea is to wake children before the urge to urinate strikes, in the hope that they are then able to make it to the bathroom in time. There are drawbacks with the use of any alarm system, however. Some children are such deep sleepers that they merely shut off the alarm and return to sleep before becoming sufficiently aroused to leave the bed. The only people who are awakened, then, are the concerned parents. And the relapse rate of alarm systems is also fairly high.

Drug therapy may be useful, but only in a small percentage of cases and for very brief periods of time. For example, imipramine (marketed as Tofranil), considered the drug of choice, can be used to prevent bed-wetting on a short-term basis—say, when the child plans to attend an overnight camp or visit grandparents for a week. Knowing that bed-wetting will not become an issue during such finite periods can work wonders for the child's self-esteem. The drug also appears to have a beneficial effect on bladder muscle tone. Imipramine will work only for a short time, however; it is merely a remedy, not a cure. Another drawback is that its use should be restricted to older children or adolescents. And like many drugs, it poses the risk of side effects, including changes in blood pressure or heart rate, especially if taken in high doses. It may even cause a degree of wakefulness—which in this case is relatively desirable, since the child is thus more likely to exercise conscious control over urination. However, the rate of relapse after the drug is discontinued is high.

Another drug called desmopressin was recently studied as a possible long-term approach; some experts believed that enuresis might not recur after a course of desmopressin therapy, in contrast to imipramine therapy. Efficacy of desmopressin, however, was found to be limited. A drug called amantadine hydrochloride is also being studied for possible use in controlling bedwetting. Generally, though, the use of drugs, especially in children, poses a number of problems in addition to side effects and expense. There have been reports of unexpected deaths of children treated for bed-wetting with tricyclic antidepressants. As a rule, then, I refrain from recommending drug strategies, especially when the success of other approaches has been so clearly demonstrated.

In a very small number of cases surgery may be needed to correct or eliminate an abnormality in the urinary system, such as an obstruction of some kind or a malformation in the bladder. For example, the ureter (the tube that conveys urine from the kidney to the bladder) may be ectopic—that is, it may open out somewhere inside the body other than the bladder wall. A diverticulum (pouch) may develop in the urethra—the urinary passage from the bladder to the outside of the body. In such cases urine collects in the pouch and may be released at night. Some children are born with epispadias, a congenital defect in which the upper wall of the urethra is missing. Males are more likely to exhibit this condition, which causes the urethra to appear as an external, unclosed groove along the top of the penis. In females epispadias takes the form of a fissure in the upper wall of the urethra.

The most effective strategy is likely to be one that combines a variety of these approaches. However, I usually caution parents that even if the strategy works four out of five times, they will find attaining 100 percent success to be a slow and trying process. Again, patience, awareness, sensitivity, and time are the most important elements in helping a child overcome a problem with bed-wetting.

OTHER FORMS OF PARASOMNIA

Bruxism is the technical name for nocturnal teeth grinding. (Daytime, conscious grinding of the jaws is a different behavioral disorder and is given the name bruxomania.) As bed partners of "bruxers" know all too well, this disorder is accompanied by a loud grating or clicking sound. Bruxism, often associated with body movements and partial arousal from sleep, usually occurs in Stage 2 sleep or after the completion of a REM episode as the sleeper returns to the start of the sleep cycle. Bruxers may perceive overall sleep as lighter and less restorative. Victims usually have no awareness that they are grinding their teeth; however, they may wake in the morning complaining of aching jaws. Their dentists may also notice tooth wear or damage to soft tissues. Incidence of bruxism is about equally divided between males and females. Estimates vary, but some authorities believe that between 5 and 10 percent of children and between 5 and 21 percent of adults grind their teeth in their sleep; the incidence declines with age.

The cause of this parasomnia is unknown. A combination of a malformed jaw and some kind of psychological stimulus—usually anxiety—is often involved. Missing or oversized teeth, or teeth that have not been properly cared for, may contribute to the problem. Stress is a likely factor in many cases. As you have no doubt experienced firsthand, one of the first ways in which stress affects your body is in a tightening of the jaw muscles. Electromyographic studies by sleep laboratories confirm that incidents of bruxism occur following stressful or fatiguing days. An oral fixation or some kind of neurological disorder similar to epilepsy may also be at work.

Effective options for managing bruxism are few. There is no specific drug targeted to address the problem, although benzodiazepines such as clonazepam may have some limited value. Other approaches involve hypnosis, autosuggestion, oral surgery, muscle relaxation exercises, aversion therapy, or biofeedback. Perhaps the strategy most likely to succeed is use of a mouth guard. Your dentist can advise you about the types of guards available.

Head Banging is a parasomnia that takes the form of rhythmic to-and-fro rocking of the head or body. This behavior, which usually begins in early childhood and disappears by adolescence, occurs in Stages 1 and 2 of the sleep cycle and stops by the time the sleeper reaches Stages 3 and 4. Although some head bangers may continue to rock for up to two hours after they fall asleep, they seem to demonstrate no further signs or symptoms on waking.

As is the case with many sleep mysteries, no cause of head banging has been firmly identified. Epilepsy has been ruled out; other theories include a variety of organic, social, and psychiatric factors—among them low IQ, understimulation, stress, maternal neglect, and excessive physical restraint. Typically, however, a head banger will demonstrate none of these problems.

About the only therapeutic option available for head banging is the use of low-dose benzodiazepines, such as oxazepam. The number of body movements will drop, but usually the patient develops a tolerance to the drug within one to four weeks, rendering it ineffective. Anticonvulsants such as phenytoin (sold as Dilantin) don't help either.

Sleep Epilepsy—seizures that occur primarily or exclusively at night—is found in about 45 percent of all epileptics. (Another 21 percent experience seizures at night as well as during the day, while the rest are affected only during daytime hours.) Organic brain disease accounts for about one in four cases of sleep epilepsy (but only about one in ten cases of waking epilepsy). Sleep epilepsy is more common in children than adults; in severe cases, a child may experience up to a hundred seizures a night. Unlike many other parasomnias, seizure disorders will not vanish with time; they require careful medical attention.

Certain types of seizures occur at specific stages in the sleep cycle, thus disrupting sleep in a number of different ways. In turn, arousal from sleep, such as the arousal that occurs at the end of a ninety-minute sleep cycle, can trigger other kinds of epileptic phenomena. Nocturnal circadian rhythms, including hormonal secretion, cerebral blood flow, body temperature, water and electrolyte excretion, and cortisol level, may also play a role in triggering nighttime seizures.

In diagnosis, it is important—and also very difficult—to distinguish sleep epilepsy from a number of other sleep disturbances, such as nocturnal myoclonus or bruxism. Even careful monitoring by a sleep laboratory and analysis of EEG tracings can be misleading. Treatment of epilepsy usually involves the use of anticonvulsive medications. Unfortunately, some research indicates that such drugs can further disrupt the sleep of epileptics.

Timing of administration (i.e., taking the drug late in the evening rather than in the morning) may help minimize this disruption.

Sleep Paralysis may be a factor in up to 50 percent of cases of narcolepsy. Occasionally, however, it can affect otherwise healthy individuals, perhaps arising as a dysfunction of the mechanism that inhibits muscle function during REM sleep. Sleep paralysis is sometimes a genetic trait, inherited from the mother, which occurs in several members of the family and is not accompanied by other symptoms. It may also be associated with obstructive sleep apnea and is an occasional feature of the Pickwickian syndrome. In some cases it occurs by itself, with no other detectable sleep abnormalities, or it may be associated with severe endogenous depression. The odds are about even that you will experience at least one episode of sleep paralysis in your lifetime.

The paralysis can be terrifying, especially when first experienced: Victims are suddenly unable to move and may feel that they are suffocating. Although usually conscious, they may slide between sleep and dreaming states, losing track of time and reality. Their hearts race, their pupils dilate, they sweat. In time, however, many patients learn that the paralysis is blessedly brief and largely benign, and thus they simply lie in bed waiting for it to pass. In each patient, attacks usually occur at the same time of night, although this time may be the beginning, middle, or end of sleep.

Earlier I described one technique for ending the paralysis, which involves progressive muscle movements starting with the eyes (see page 144). Antidepressive drugs such as imipramine, desipramine, and especially clomipramine may help prevent attacks. This preventive effect usually occurs within a day or two— a much shorter time than the one to eight weeks required for these drugs to work when used to improve mood.

Nocturnal penile tumescence (NPT), or sleeping erections, are normal and universal in men, occurring usually during the REM cycle. In rare cases, however, the erections can be prolonged and painful, resulting in disturbed sleep. If the problem is severe, there may be several awakenings during the night; it may take a few minutes for the erection to subside. Fortunately, men with painful NPT do not usually suffer sexual dysfunction during their waking hours. (NPT is different from priapism, in which erections do not subside.) In some cases, NPT may stem from high blood pressure or other vascular disease; if so, treatment for hypertension may help. Another approach involves waking the patient at the onset of REM sleep, which may work by preventing the physical changes in blood circulation that accompany the REM cycle, or by preventing dreams that produce erections. Occasionally, however, NPT may be caused by a penile disorder such as phimosis (constricture of the foreskin which prevents it from retracting over the head of the penis) or Peyronie's disease (a thickening and contracting of fibers surrounding the main body of the penis).

Sleeptalking At some point in our lives, most of us have been told about (and probably embarrassed by) our nighttime mumblings. The content of these conversations depends on what stage of sleep you have reached. If you talk during a NREM period, for example, your remarks will appear unemotional and will focus on trivial matters. Surprisingly, people are less prone to talk during the dream-filled REM phase. When they do, their remarks are much more likely to be tinged with emotion and will usually be related in some way to the content of their dreams. I remember a case in which the husband complained that his wife's incessant nocturnal chatter kept him awake at night. I suggested that the next time this happened he try to enter the conversation gently by saying, "Please stop talking now and go to sleep." The patient later reported that he had followed my advice and told me—to my surprise, I must admit—that his wife had replied sweetly, "Okay!" then turned over and kept quiet at night for weeks afterward.

Other Conditions

I have already mentioned other conditions that can affect the quality of sleep. They include pain, cluster headaches, gastrointestinal disturbances, and cardiovascular disorders. Proper medical attention, under the guidance of a physician, is the best way to minimize the impact these other conditions have on your sleep. Usually, sleep will improve when these conditions are managed properly.

In the next chapter, I will present some straightforward strategies that you can use to help get a good night's sleep— strategies that, by themselves, will often provide the relief you seek.

8

Help Yourself to a Good Night's Sleep

Throughout this book I've touched briefly on some of the treatment options available for a variety of sleep disorders. In this chapter I'll focus on the many steps you can take on your own to improve your sleeping habits and patterns. These strategies—which for the most part are just therapeutic doses of simple common sense—are easy to implement, demand no investment other than a little time and thought, and have helped thousands of poor sleepers.

You may notice some improvement soon after adopting these approaches. A more lasting impact on your insomnia, however, will take time; a lifetime of bad sleep habits can't be unlearned overnight. Plan on allowing about four to five weeks before expecting to see results. Without knowing you personally, I can't recommend any specific strategy. No single technique works for everyone, nor does one necessarily hold any particular value over another. Look over the options carefully, decide which ones apply to you, and gradually, over a period of a few weeks, try the ones you feel are appropriate or have the greatest chance of success.

However, if after reading the previous chapters you suspect there may be some medical basis for your insomnia, I urge you to see a physician as soon as possible. I also caution you that more difficult or intractable cases require the attention of sleep experts who, after a careful assessment of your condition, may recommend a combination of therapies, possibly including psychological counseling and the use of drugs. I'll outline the options for professional intervention in the following chapter.

LIFESTYLE

The process of falling asleep begins the minute you awaken in the morning. By that I mean that insomnia is not a problem that just crops up suddenly at night. The way you live every waking moment—your thoughts, your habits, the way you interact with other people, even your taste in home decor—affects your ability to sleep. Obviously, you can't abuse your body and your brain through a deficient diet, insufficient exercise, excessive emotional stress, and an onslaught of caffeine or alcohol and expect to get a good night's sleep. Too much or too little of anything—food, stimulation, sleep—can be harmful. Generally the simplest way to bring about improvements in sleep is to adopt the policy on which ancient Greek civilization was founded: "Moderation in all things." Or, as one sleep expert put it, "The best recipe for sleeping well is living well."

Here, then, are some of the key ingredients of that recipe.

Limit Your Intake of Caffeine

Caffeine, nicotine, and alcohol are the three drugs that most commonly contribute to insomnia. You should think of caffeine as a drug of the stimulant class, although it is of course much less powerful than other stimulants such as amphetamines or cocaine. Chemically caffeine resembles uric acid, an endogenous or "built-in" compound found in the blood of primates but not other vertebrates. Some researchers believe that our bodies' supply of uric acid may act as a form of "natural caffeine" in providing continuous nervous stimulation, which in turn may help account for our higher intelligence as well as such traits as drive and leadership.

Common Sources of Caffeine

Product		Caffeine
Instant coffee	(1 cup)	66 milligrams (mg)
Coffee—percolated	"	110 mg
Coffee—drip brewed	"	146 mg
Tea—brewed 1 minute	"	25 mg
Tea—Brewed 5 minutes	"	46 mg
Cocoa	"	13 mg
Jolt Cola	(12-ounce can)	120 mg
Coca-Cola	"	60 mg
Dr Pepper	"	60 mg
Tab	"	49 mg
Pepsi Cola	"	43 mg
Chocolate bar	(approx. 2 ounces)	25 mg

Nonprescription stimulants:

Vivarin	200 mg
Caffedrine	200 mg
No Doz	100 mg
Pre-mens Forte	100 mg
Aqua-Ban (over-the-counter diuretic)	100 mg

Nonprescription medications:

Excedrin	64 mg
Vanquish	32 mg
Anacin	32 mg
Emprin	32 mg
Midol	32 mg
Dristan	16 mg

The amount of caffeine contained in even one cup of coffee is enough to affect the way your brain and body operate. Many people depend on their morning dose to "get their thoughts flowing." But caffeine stimulates the flow of electrical signals to the muscles as well, which is why you may feel a caffeine "buzz" or notice a slight tremor in your hands or fingers. With larger doses your heart rate and respiration speed up. You may even hear a ringing in your ears.

Of course, many people tolerate, and in fact seek, the relatively mild agitation caffeine provides. Habitual coffee drinkers usually have no trouble falling asleep, even if they drink coffee in the evening, although their sleep cycle may be disturbed to some extent. Lighter sleepers, however, may toss and turn if they have just a single cup with dinner.

There are a number of steps you can take to restrict your caffeine intake. First, write down the amount of caffeine you ingest in the course of a day. Just seeing the total may help make you aware of the extent to which caffeine may be contributing to your insomnia.

Obviously, switching to decaffeinated coffee or tea can make a big difference. In response to public concern over caffeine intake, tea makers today are producing a variety of herbal and flavored teas, ranging from almond and apple to cranberry and cinnamon. Such products provide a soothing and tasty alternative to caffeinated drinks while satisfying the desire to drink a hot liquid. Most restaurants have become aware that many customers are watching their caffeine intake, and have made flavorful brewed decaf available.

Some people, of course, find it virtually impossible to do without chocolate, but a number of caffeine-free snacks, such as carob- or yogurt-covered peanuts, may provide an adequate substitute. (Such treats do contribute calories you may not want, however—remember to practice moderation.)

If you can't go cold turkey and eliminate caffeine entirely, start by cutting back. Look at your total caffeine intake and try reducing it by a significant amount—a half or even a quarter—over a period of two weeks. Recently one coffee maker introduced a form of "lite" coffee containing only half the usual amount of caffeine. If you still have trouble falling asleep, keep cutting back as much as possible. Use a smaller coffee cup or limit the time of consumption. For example, make it a rule to drink no coffee after, say, six o'clock or, better yet, after your noontime meal.

You may need to enlist the help of others in your crusade. Ask your mate to reinforce your efforts by not requesting coffee with dinner or by switching to decaffeinated coffee. If you work in an office that supplies coffee as a "perk" (no pun intended) ask that decaf be provided as an option.

Stop Smoking

Nicotine—the stimulating element of cigarette smoke—is absorbed through the mucous linings of the mouth and lungs, where it passes into the blood and circulates to the brain. There it triggers a variety of nervous system responses, among them alterations in the width of the airways in the lungs. Eventually nicotine reaches the hypothalamus, the control center of a number of vital functions, including appetite. Nicotine can also affect the cardiovascular system by causing tachycardia (excessively fast heartbeat), increased cardiac output, constriction of the blood vessels, and elevated blood pressure. Such stimulating effects, as we have seen, can disrupt sleep. What's more, nicotine is the cause of the craving for cigarettes; this craving can in itself wake smokers, who may then be unable to return to sleep until they have had a smoke.

Quitting smoking, of course, provides benefits beyond simply improving sleep. It is notoriously difficult to do, but, fortunately, there are a number of methods available that can help, ranging from aversion therapy to hypnosis. If possible, seek the advice of your physician, who may be able to suggest an approach and can help reinforce your efforts. Much publicity has been given recently to nicotine gums, available by prescription, which satisfy the urge for nicotine and reduce the desire for cigarettes. Such gums, however, still introduce nicotine into the body and consequently may not help your sleep patterns.

I should also note that some insomniacs, if deprived of caffeine or nicotine, may become agitated unless they get a "fix"; in these extreme cases, coffee and cigarettes paradoxically provide some measure of relaxation.

Moderate Your Intake of Alcohol

I experience a small shudder whenever I hear patients say they "always have a little nightcap" to help them sleep. As we have seen, the relaxed feeling induced by alcohol does lead to drowsiness in the short term. But after the alcohol has been absorbed—about five hours into the night—there is a withdrawal effect which fragments, lightens, and otherwise disrupts sleep. It is during this phase that troubling dreams, previously suppressed, may attack the sleeper. Eventually drinkers develop a tolerance, meaning that more and more liquor is needed to achieve the same drowsiness. This in turn leads to more withdrawal effect and chronic sleep fragmentation—another of the many sleep-disturbing vicious circles we have discussed.

Physiologically alcohol causes the oropharyngeal muscles (located in the mouth and throat region) to relax, represses the mechanism that drives respiratory function, and reduces the ability of the body to awaken. Thus a nightcap can cause, or at least aggravate, sleep apnea, especially central sleep apnea. Drinking reduces the level of oxygen in the blood, which in turn leads to increased snoring and the accompanying risks I have already described, including asphyxiation. Some researchers are even convinced that alcohol-related oxygen starvation is an important cause of brain damage.

If you are in the habit of taking alcohol at bedtime, try to stop. At least limit the amount to less than an ounce, or restrict drinking to a period of an hour or two in the early evening. If you find that none of these steps is possible for you, your problem may be deeper than simple insomnia. You may have a drinking problem and should seek professional help and group support to overcome it.

Use Drugs Only When Necessary

A number of prescription and nonprescription medications can contribute to sleeping problems. Along with their beneficial therapeutic effects, asthma preparations, amphetamines, and steroids can stimulate body organs and metabolic processes, thus disrupting normal activity, including the functioning of circadian rhythms. Sleep medications themselves, such as barbiturates, ethchlorvynol (sold as Placidyl), and glutethimide (Doriden), as well as such antianxiety agents as meprobamate (a tranquilizer sold under a variety of names including Equanil and Miltown), can create tolerance and cause withdrawal symptoms to arise during the night, in some cases leading to disrupted sleep after only two weeks. Daytime drowsiness may be a side effect of sedatives, hypnotics, anticonvulsants, antihypertensives, antihistamines, and antidepressants, particularly if such drugs are taken during the daylight hours.

Before embarking upon or changing any drug regimen, *consult with your physician.* When you do, it is imperative that you inform the doctor of all drugs you are currently using—including any illegal ones such as cocaine or marijuana—in order to supply a true drug profile. Sometimes a patient may be taking a drug unnecessarily, long after the condition has resolved, simply because he or she did not return to the physician for a follow-up examination. If so, it may be a relatively easy matter to terminate use of the drug. The physician may also have suggestions about altering dosage strength, timing of administration, or switching to related drugs or other formulations in order to improve therapeutic benefit while reducing the actual amount of drug taken.

Eat Right to Sleep Right

For our purposes, the old adage "You are what you eat" should be rewritten "You sleep what you eat." There are a number of dietary strategies that may improve your ability to get a good night's rest. A high-carbohydrate diet, for example, serves to facilitate sleep. So too does consumption of food that elevates levels of a substance called tryptophan, an amino acid involved in the production of the neurotransmitter serotonin. Serotonin, in turn, facilitates sleep. Research indicates that a diet rich in carbohydrates, or a balanced combination of carbohydrates and fats, may lead to elevated serotonin and will thus improve sleep. (Protein-rich foods do not boost tryptophan levels as much as carbohydrates.)

Among the foods that are naturally high in tryptophan are dairy products including whole or skim milk, cheddar cheese, cottage cheese, and eggs; meats, including roast beef, ground beef, sirloin steak, loin pork chops, fresh (not canned) ham, veal cutlet, lamb chops, and turkey; and nuts.

Tryptophan Guidelines

It has been shown that the use of tryptophan can reduce the time before sleep onset by as much as 50 percent—say, from

Carbohydrates include:

* Breads
* Cereals
* Grains
* Fruits
* Pasta
* Potatoes
* Rice
* Corn

Foods that are high in fat are:

* Cheese
* Cream
* Ice cream
* Sour cream
* Mayonnaise
* Nuts (macadamias, pecans, hickory nuts, peanuts)
* Peanut butter

twenty minutes to ten minutes. A well-balanced diet, including reasonable portions of the foods listed above, will usually provide enough tryptophan to maintain sleep.

Since one of the main sources of tryptophan is milk, there is wisdom in the folk remedy of drinking warm milk at bedtime. Research suggests that malted milk may be even more effective than regular milk in helping facilitate sleep. However, some experts caution that the therapeutic dose of tryptophan is the equivalent of six glasses of milk, and thus a single glass may not be adequate. And be careful: overconsumption of milk poses other dietary hazards, including high cholesterol levels which may lead to heart disease.

Pure tryptophan is available from health food stores and drugstores in capsule or tablet form as a dietary supplement. One commonly recommended regimen is 1 to 2 grams of tryptophan taken about forty-five minutes before bedtime. Such a regimen may work for only three nights in a row; however, by then you may have established an adequate sleeping pattern.

As with any therapy, proceed with caution. Some people report nausea and vomiting after taking high doses (up to 10 grams) of tryptophan.

Other Dietary Strategies

The goal of any diet should be to provide adequate nutrition based on a balanced selection of various kinds of foods. To maintain nutritional balance and caloric intake, some experts suggest you shift consumption of carbohydrates from the morning and noon meals to the nighttime meal. And, of course, it's sensible to eat moderately and to establish regular mealtimes. Many people have found that drinking chamomile tea in the evening promotes sleep.

In addition to the composition of your diet, the timing of your meals may affect your sleep. For example, try to eat meals on a regular schedule, so that your body knows what to expect. If your circadian rhythms are cued to receive dinner every evening at six, your various digestive mechanisms will be activated automatically at that time. If food does not subsequently arrive or is delayed for two or three hours, the timing of the mechanisms is disrupted, with consequences that can disturb your sleep.

Don't go to bed hungry, but remember that eating a big meal even an hour or two before bedtime can be a problem. For example, a full stomach triggers various systems in the body to go into high gear; your heart works harder and the digestive system churns out digestive juices. Body temperature rises as a consequence of all this activity whereas, normally, temperature would drop as part of the circadian dewaking process. As a rule of thumb, then, remember: the *later* the meal, the *lighter* the meal.

Techniques from other countries include:

* Ginseng tea and dried orange juice mixed with honey (China)
* An apple, chewed slowly before bedtime (England)
* Mushrooms (Pueblo Indians)
* Pollen cake (Burma)

Exercise

Regular vigorous exercises produces a world of benefits, improvements in your sleep being but one. No single specific program of exercise is right for everyone at every stage of life. Many people feel that active walking and swimming are the best strategies, producing the best results with the minimum risk of strain or injury. Your own exercise regimen must suit your abilities and lifestyle and should be undertaken only after consulting with a physician.

With regard to sleep, the *timing* of your exercise is most critical. Remember, exercise taken late in the evening—beyond, say, eight or nine o'clock—can raise body temperature to the point where falling asleep becomes difficult. And such competitive sports as racquetball may stimulate your system so much that relaxing and dropping off to sleep become problematic.

Exercising in the morning has the least effect on your sleeping patterns, while afternoon exercise has been found to increase the deeper sleep stages that occur in the first half of the night. If you are unable to take your exercise soon after rising, then try to do so during a noontime break. Some of my patients have discov-

---

EXERCISE TIPS

* *Get medical advice* before beginning an exercise program (especially if you are out of shape).
* Plan on at least twenty minutes of exercise three times a week; some experts feel this time should be extended to between thirty minutes and an hour five to seven times a week.
* Warm up before beginning; cool down after stopping.
* Exercise should be vigorous and continuous to the point where it produces muscle fatigue. It is really only *after* exercise, during the process of muscle rest and rebuilding, that improvements in tone and strength occur.
* Sex does not count as bedtime exercise. (However, healthy, active, satisfying sex—as many people have discovered—is conducive to a good night's sleep.)

ered that exercise during the afternoon can also be a very beneficial way to circumvent the temptation to nap; it keeps them from robbing themselves of precious nighttime sleep. Other good times to exercise are just after work and before dinner. (Working out on a full stomach is not advisable.) In any case, your regimen should be completed at least four hours before bedtime.

Be aware that the improvement in sleep due to exercise may be long in coming, perhaps weeks or months. A heavy workout one day will not automatically deepen sleep that night.

Put Your Mind to Rest

As we have seen, emotional and mental turbulence can disrupt the process of sleep. The death of a spouse, child, relative, or close friend is an obvious and understandable cause of anguish. In addition, stress-related insomnia can be triggered by a disruption or a change in virtually any aspect of your daily life, including the following.

* Marital: marriage, separation, divorce, reconciliation
* Domestic: birth of a child, moving to a new location, child leaving home, conflict between spouses or siblings
* Financial: sudden loss (or increase) of income, unexpected expenses
* Employment: new job, promotion, loss of job, turmoil or discord within your company, pressure, competition
* Health: illness, injury, or hospitalization, your own or that of someone in the family
* Social: retirement, involvement in a legal conflict, jail term

Certain behavior patterns or emotional habits can also affect your ability to get a good night's rest.

* Feelings of anger, frustration, hostility, competitiveness, aggression
* Repression or suppression of such feelings
* Inability to relax
* Tendency to ruminate, especially while in bed

* Sexual fears or frustrations
* Other fears, especially of darkness or death

If you are unable to sleep, take some time to look carefully at your situation. Think back over the last few weeks, or the past year, and determine if any events or feelings similar to the ones mentioned above might be playing some role in your current sleep difficulty. Sometimes just becoming aware of a problem, acknowledging its impact or realizing a pattern of events, can be the first step in resolving the crisis. Fortunately, much of the sleeplessness arising from such situations is transient and will pass within a few days or a few weeks. As a physician, I am constantly amazed at the human ability to absorb the blows dealt out by life in the modern world, then to bounce back within a relatively short period. If you experience a traumatic change in your life, one that disturbs your ability to sleep, rest assured that in most cases time will provide the cure as you learn to recognize, adjust to, and cope with your new circumstances.

As we have seen, in some cases insomnia may stem from a deep-seated fear of death. Sleep is sometimes referred to poetically as "the little death." The comparison is apt: when we sleep, we enter a dark environment, lie down, close our eyes, and surrender conscious control of our senses to a mysterious and little-understood force.

If you feel a sense of dread as bedtime approaches or as you enter the bedroom, consider your feelings about death and dying. You may wish to discuss these feelings with a professional counselor. There are also a few simple things you can do yourself to make your bedroom more attractive and less "cryptlike." Use of a night-light can help. Not only is the presence of light reassuring as you fall asleep, it can help orient you and provide comfort should you awaken during the night. Also, make your bedroom a warm and inviting place. Don't be hesitant to wear luxurious and comfortable sleep garb or to indulge in beautiful and sensual bedclothes. If you find silk sheets to be the height of luxury, and can sleep on them without slipping out onto the floor, by all means use them. Make sure your bedroom is clean, uncluttered, and decorated with objects or artwork you find attractive and appealing. Even the use of mild incense or air scents may improve the ambience. I'll have more to say about the bedroom environment later in this chapter.

Often the mental and emotional causes of sleep disturbance are deeply rooted and need more aggressive treatment than the simple steps I've just described. For example, earlier we discussed the role depression can play in causing insomnia. If you suspect you suffer from depression, you may find the following exercise helpful.

DEPRESSION EVALUATION

Read the following pairs of statements. Rank yourself on a scale of 1 to 10, depending on the degree to which one of the statements accurately describes your feelings or your situation.

I must emphasize that this exercise is provided only *as one potential means of assistance in your health evaluation. It is not intended to replace, supplement, or contrast with any other self-assessment depression scale. Furthermore, under no circumstances, should this exercise be used to replace the evaluation of a medical professional. If you think you may be suffering from depression, regardless of your ranking on the exercise, you should* always *seek professional help.*

Rank

1. I cry often. . . . . I seldom cry. _____

2. Small things upset . . . . . Small things don't _____
   me easily.   bother me.

3. I don't remember things . . . . My mind is _____
   as easily as I used to.   as sharp as ever.

4. I find it hard to . . . . I can usually _____
   concentrate on   concentrate when I
   anything.   need to.

5. I feel restless. . . . . I feel relaxed. _____

6. I'd rather stay home. . . . .   I enjoy getting out _____
                                  and being with people.

7. I don't like to try . . . . I like to try _____
   new things.   new things.

8. I tend to dwell . . . . I don't usually dwell _____
   on certain thoughts.   on certain thoughts.

9. I feel worthless. . . . . I feel worthy. _____

10. I feel hopeless. . . . . I feel hopeful. _____

11. I feel helpless. . . . . I feel in control. _____

12. I am easily bored. . . . . I have many interests. _____

13. My life is empty. . . . . My life is full. _____

14. I worry about . . . . I look forward to _____
    the future.   the future.

15. I dwell on the . . . . I don't dwell on the _____
    past.   past.

16. I feel something bad . . . I feel something good _____
    is going to happen   is going to happen
    to me.   to me.

17. I can't get started . . . . I take on new _____
    on things.   projects willingly.

18. Everyone else is better . . . . I think I'm _____
    off than I am.   pretty well off.

19. I don't pursue . . . . I keep up with _____
    my old hobbies.   my hobbies.

20. I am dissatisfied . . . . I am satisfied _____
    with my life.   with my life.

21. It's difficult to . . . . I make decisions _____
    make decisions.   quickly and easily.

22. I don't look . . . . I look _____
    forward to morning.   forward to morning.

23. I have no energy. . . . . . . I am full of energy. _____

24. My life is dull. . . . . My life is exciting. _____

25. I am never . . . . I am always _____
    in good spirits.   in good spirits.
                                               TOTAL

Add up the numbers in the Rank column and note the total. A score of less than 125 indicates that you *may* be suffering from some form of clinical depression and may wish to consider seeking professional help. But remember, regardless of your score, if you think you might be suffering from depression, you should seek professional help.

Cut Out Naps

Granted, naps have their place. When properly used, naps by whatever name—catnaps, forty winks, quick snoozes—can refresh you and restore your energy level. Sometimes defined as "rests of short periods involving unconsciousness but not pajamas," naps offer a temporary escape from the pressures of the day, allowing you to "check out" for a short time and return to the battle with renewed strength. It's possible, too, that an occasional nap can help clear the brain, enabling you to formulate solutions to problems that elude your mind in its waking, and frequently chaotic, state. In fact, one leading businessman recommends "businessman's naps," claiming they are one secret of his success.

Recognizing that people's energy levels almost universally dip following lunch, a number of societies have ordained the nap as a respected feature of their culture. Perhaps best known is the siesta, prominent in tropical climates, where activity drops as the sun rises. As Noel Coward's song states, only "mad dogs and Englishmen" would be foolish enough to go out into the noonday sun in these parts of the globe. Far from being a sign of laziness or indolence, the siesta is a reasonable adaptation to an inescapable feature of the environment. But midday naps are not unique to the tropics. In Vienna people enjoy a respite called the *Mittagsschläfchen* (or "little midday sleep"). In Oslo too people nap, despite the fact that their winter nights are so long.

For people with nighttime insomnia, however, naps are a source of trouble. As we have seen, your body is primed to sleep a certain amount over a twenty-four-hour period. The amount can vary, but any naps you take should be thought of as robbing time from nocturnal sleep. Thus, you may feel the need to grab an hour's shut-eye after lunch, but you should be prepared to wake up an hour earlier the following morning. Even if you manage to stay in bed as long as usual, you are likely to perceive your sleep as lighter and less restful. Lighter sleep can then lead to excessive daytime sleepiness, in turn causing a stronger desire to nap and leading again to disrupted sleep the following night. Such a vicious circle serves only to entrench the insomnia.

Sleepy people tend to spend extra time in bed without actually enjoying restorative sleep. By lolling in bed they are prone to random napping—ten minutes here, five minutes there—a process that can create an irregular circadian sleep-wake cycle. When that cycle is disrupted, it can throw the hormone and body temperature rhythms out of whack, resulting in a more serious case of insomnia.

In some cases, such as narcolepsy or rare cases of severe insomnia, naps can be helpful or therapeutic. But if you have difficulty falling asleep, or if you wake too early in the morning, or if you are sleepy during the day, you should structure your sleep so as to prevent, or at least minimize, naps. One way to do so is to undertake some other activity as a substitute for napping. Reading can work, but it can also be soporific. So many people read to fall asleep that during the day the very act of reading becomes a sort of Pavlovian trigger for sleepiness. Better, perhaps, to take a brisk walk. Fresh air and exercise can be invigorating, and can help supply exercise which in turn will help you sleep better that night. You may be able to schedule your work activities so that certain physical or otherwise more stimulating tasks can be done during the hour or so following lunch: try returning phone calls, for example, instead of reviewing budgetary figures.

If you must nap, there are some steps you can take to lessen the damage. For example, try resting while sitting in a chair, not lying down. Some researchers also feel that the ninety-minute sleep cycles we experience at night are reflected in similar ninety-minute cycles of energy and body activity during the day. These waking cycles tend to coincide with unexplained variations in our attention span, sudden unprovoked sexual arousal, or a momentary lapse into fantasy and daydreaming. This circadian dip in energy level, as I have mentioned, is also thought to account for the increase in auto accidents at certain times of day. Some experts suggest that if you must nap, the nap should last as long as one complete sleep cycle—in other words, from sixty to ninety minutes. In addition, plan on cutting back your nighttime sleep by the equivalent amount.

Take Control of Your Schedule

The best way to manage sleep is to set a strict schedule for going to bed and rising in the morning, and stick to it. I'll offer more details on this approach shortly. First, though, with respect to scheduling, I want to remind you again that if your job or lifestyle requires you to travel a great deal, it will pay you to review the strategies for anticipating and managing the effects of jet lag outlined in Chapter 2.

Also, if you are required to work different shifts and you experience trouble sleeping, there are steps you can take to lessen the impact. As I mentioned earlier, you may be able to negotiate with your employer to use a rotation that moves work shifts forward—that is, from daytime to evening to night shifts—over a period of about four weeks, in order to accommodate the natural circadian cycles. If such flexibility is not possible or desirable in your situation, at least try to eat your meals at the same time, and try to sleep during the same four-hour period, every day. Of course, you should try to create a bedroom atmosphere that is conducive to sleep: minimize noise and light by using heavy shades and curtains or other soundproofing techniques. Avoid stimulant drugs, including coffee, especially in the hours before bedtime. And make it easy on yourself. If at all possible, avoid sudden changes in schedule on weekends. Enlist your family's understanding and help in relieving your burden by adjusting their lives to match yours where possible. For example, don't plan family outings or home projects for the first thing Saturday morning; aim for an after-lunch event. Such efforts may involve sacrifices for all concerned but will pay off by providing more relaxed, productive, or rewarding hours in return.

THE BEDROOM ENVIRONMENT

Up to now, my recommendations have focused on changes you may be able to effect in your style of living in order to improve your style of sleeping. In addition, there may be some practical steps you can take to make your sleeping quarters more conducive to a good night's rest.

To start, take a good look at your bedroom or sleeping area. What does it say about you and your habits? Is the space dedicated to sleep, or is it a sort of multipurpose room, serving as a combination dining room/den/entertainment center? If so, at least one cause of your insomnia may be right in front of your eyes.

Read the following survey. The answers you give to the questions may indicate that some changes are needed if you expect to sleep better in the coming weeks and years.

* Is the room quiet?
* If not, where does the noise come from? Neighbors (above, below, next door), family room, children's bedroom, outside (trains, sirens, traffic)?
* If noise penetrates, is there anything you can do to minimize it (soundproof, talk to neighbors, discipline children, etc.)?
* Is the room dark enough?
* If not, is there anything you can do to reduce penetrating light (i.e., heavier shades, curtains, awnings)?
* Is the room comfortable (adequate heat, air-conditioning, humidity)?
* Is the room large enough to accommodate you, your bed partner, furnishings, closets, and knickknacks?
* Is the room cluttered or tidy, busy or sparse?
* Is it decorated in a pleasing way? Are the walls painted in bright colors and bedecked with stimulating artwork?

* Do you use the room exclusively for sleep, or is it also used as a desk/work area, for personal entertainment (television, VCR, music system) or other purposes (socializing, hobbies, etc.)?
* Is your bed large enough for your needs? Is the layout of furniture, doors, and windows agreeable?
* Are your bed furnishings (pillows, blankets, mattress) comfortable?

Depending on your answers to these questions, some improvements in your sleeping space may be in order.

Use the Bedroom for Sleep (And Sex)

By this I simply mean that, with the exception of sexual intercourse, other activities often conducted in the bedroom may be incompatible with sleep. For example, if it is your practice to pay bills at the bedroom desk before turning in, you may find yourself more likely to lie awake worrying about your ability to meet your financial obligations. If you watch a scary movie on your bedroom VCR, you may become too stimulated to drop off, or your dreams may be filled with frightening images. Similarly, reading a mystery novel in bed may entice you to stay up past your usual sleep time and cause your brain to keep working over an unsolved puzzle. Lying in bed chewing over the problems of the day, or using the bed as the site of arguments or emotional discussions with your mate, can cause the act of retiring to become laden with unpleasant associations.

If you engage in these activities and have trouble sleeping, try shifting them to another location. Write checks at the dinner table, for instance; read books on the living room couch. Avoid bedtime entertainments that can agitate or disturb your peace of mind. And confine marital or other squabbles to other rooms of the house. Don't let your daytime troubles disrupt your nighttime rest.

Obviously financial constraints require that some people use their sleeping space for other purposes as well. Many individuals in these circumstances turn their beds into couches during the day or use their living rooms as their bedrooms. Short of moving to other quarters, many apartment-dwellers are limited in their options for designing optimum sleeping space. Consequently they must focus on other ways to make the bed area more conducive to adequate rest, such as using a loft or Murphy bed.

Control Your Physical Sleep Environment

You will spend a third of your life, an amount of time measured in decades, in your bed—far more time, obviously, than that spent at your oak dining table or your crushed velour reclining chair. I would advise you, therefore, to buy the best, most comfortable bed you can afford, in terms of space as well as dollars. If there isn't room for you and your bed partner (and your child, if that is your choice), the remaining two-thirds of your day could be miserable. Be sure your mattress is of adequate firmness. A mattress that is too soft may collapse, making you feel as if you're sleeping on a marshmallow parked on the side of a hill. Remember the story of the princess and the pea: sometimes a lumpy mattress, or one with a broken spring, can become a royal pain.

Remember, too, that differences in the way men and women sleep can be problematic. As we've seen, men are more prone to snoring and to movement disorders, such as nocturnal myoclonus. And, of course, men generally weigh more than women; a difference of only twenty pounds can cause a trough in the bed into which the lighter partner is liable to slide. Movement by one partner is movement by both: research indicates that when one person in a bed shifts, the other is also likely to move within about half a minute and, in addition, is likely to enter a lighter stage of sleep. If such problems exist in your case, explore alternatives. For example, a number of companies offer beds with one box spring but two half-size mattresses, so that movements by one partner are less likely to affect the other.

Use A Pillow That's Right For You

If, like me, you are one of those who can't stand the stiffness and unfluffability of a foam pillow, spend the extra money and get a down pillow, one that conforms to the requirements of your head and neck. And if you are unable to find one that suits your needs, have one custom-made to your specifications. It's worth the investment. Also, if you have sleep apnea, you may find that elevating your head with two or more pillows helps alleviate the problem.

Be Sure Your Blankets and Sheets are Adequate

Such a tip seems obvious but, surprisingly, some people persist in using the wrong size sheets simply because they were a wedding gift or an inheritance from a beloved relative, or because they were on sale. Using larger-size bedclothes can do much to minimize the skirmishes fought in the nightly battle of the blankets. Torn or worn sheets, like cracked automobile windshields, will only continue to deteriorate; replace them. Many people enjoy the snuggly warmth of a thick down comforter or the luxurious pressure of a large quilt; others can't stand so much warmth or weight, preferring a lighter blanket.

Ideally, bed partners will desire the same degree and weight of bedclothes. This, however, is not always the case. For such people, an electric blanket may be the answer. I can't cite statistics, but I believe that the invention of dual-control electric blankets has saved a number of marriages in recent years. Incidentally, you may get better results if you place your electric blanket under the bottom (fitted) sheet rather than over you. Also, use of a top sheet even on warm summer nights will keep you more comfortable than no covers at all; if nothing else, the sheet will keep breezes from ruffling sensitive body hairs and disturbing your sleep.

Dress (Or Undress) for Sleep Comfort

If you find pajamas or nightshirts too confining, don't wear them. As many as 40 percent of women and 25 percent of men sleep naked, relying on sheets, blankets, and bedmates for warmth. If your feet get cold, wear socks or slipper-socks. Nightcaps (headwear, not liquor) will keep your head warm but may cause you to wake with an outrageous new hairstyle.

Keep the Room Temperature at the Right Setting

Although once they get used to it people can sleep comfortably in temperatures ranging from 50 to 90 degrees, most find a room that's somewhat on the cool side (64–66 degrees) more conducive to proper sleep. Any cooler than that, however, and you're likely to want to stay snuggled under the covers rather than hit the deck in the morning. And a room that's too warm will cause you to toss and turn more.

Use A Humidifier

Especially during the winter months, a humidifier will help alleviate the dryness in the air caused by artificial heat, and it can make snorers (and their partners) breathe easier. Recently, ultrasonic humidifiers have come onto the market which provide effective moisturizing and are virtually silent—a real asset come bedtime. If you do use a humidifier, be sure and follow the manufacturer's instructions for cleaning and maintenance. The water in a humidifier can become a breeding ground for harmful bacteria.

Turn Out the Light

Light streaming through the windows—from streetlamps, illuminated signs, neighboring buildings, or morning sun—can be an annoying cause of sleeplessness. Window shades come in a variety of opacities; judicious use of curtains can help further. Some people find that the use of facial masks or eyeshades eliminates their awareness of any ambient light. Most people, however, find that the presence of a minimum amount of light is actually reassuring and helps facilitate sleep.

Shut Out the Noise

Noise is another factor that must be controlled. Any sound greater than 70 decibels triggers a response from the nervous system: blood pressure increases and the supply of blood to the heart drops. At higher levels the pupils of the eyes dilate, even though the lids are closed. Heart rate quickens, and the respiratory muscles contract. Some people, however, are sound sleepers. Children, for example, have been found to sleep through noise levels up to 123 decibels—louder than a lawn mower and 90 decibels higher than the average background noise level during waking hours. (Of course, many parents of children who sleep poorly are convinced their offspring can wake at the sound of water dripping—in a neighbor's house.)

People usually develop a tolerance to any constant background sound (the ticking of a clock, for instance, or the whir of a generator). What's more, such tolerance appears to be selective: fathers are notorious for sleeping through the cries of their children, while mothers will be up and running with the first faint whimper. One of my fellow physicians reports that at night he will hear his paging beeper and not the children; his wife hears the children and not the beeper.

Any sudden or intermittent noise, including the hum of traffic or the buzz of a passing plane, can disrupt sleep. What's more, the disturbance will often persist even when the noise has ceased. A blaring car horn may last only a second or two, but it may take you several minutes to fall back asleep.

If noise is a problem, try to locate its source and deal with it directly. Restrict family activities in the home so as to prevent noise pollution; be sure TVs and music systems are equipped with headphones. Talk to noisy neighbors and inform them of your situation; if they prove uncooperative, don't hesitate to consult with the authorities (landlords, city managers) charged with the responsibility of maintaining the quality of living. You may not be able to convince the local airport to quit scheduling flights during your sleeping hours, but many communities have banded together to demand that their governments assess noise levels and enforce or enact flight restrictions. You may need to invest in remodeling work aimed at improving the level of sound insulation in your bedroom walls. Short of that, carpets, drapes, and acoustical ceiling tiles can reduce noise pollution to a considerable extent. Snoring is a different problem, which has been discussed elsewhere.

Techniques to mask noise can work. Recordings of natural or environmental sounds, such as ocean waves, are available. You can also buy "white noise" generators, which are nothing more than little machines that sit in a corner and hum, using noise to drown out noise. In the appropriate season fans or air conditioners can serve a similar purpose. Some people find earplugs a reasonable solution, although others find them uncomfortable or fear they may not hear the phone or the smoke detector alarm. If you want to try earplugs, you may wish to ask a doctor or pharmacist for a recommendation.

Watch Your Windows

When it comes to sleep, windows can be either a blessing or a curse. Some people insist on having fresh air stream through the room at night but can't stand the noise and light an open window admits. Window fans can help mask outside noise while circulating fresh air; large self-standing partitions may help prevent unwanted light from reaching your sleeping eyes. In some cases, simply rearranging bedroom furniture may provide the solution.

Remember That Allergies Are Nothing to Sneeze At

One other often overlooked cause of sleep disturbance is the presence of allergens in the bedroom. Be sure to keep the room clean and dusted, especially if you are prone to allergies. Don't allow smoking or pets in the bedroom. Use foam pillows if feathers make you sneeze. Also, although it should be unnecessary to say so, maintain the proper degree of cleanliness. Wash and change sheets, pillowcases, and nightclothes frequently; don't provide a hospitable environment to insects and mites.

SLEEP HYGIENE

In this context, "sleep hygiene" refers not to bodily cleanliness, although that is certainly important, but to the habits and practices involved with the actual act of going to bed. The rituals you adopt at bedtime and on rising are among the most crucial components of assuring a decent night's rest. To psychiatrists the following techniques are known as stimulus control therapies, in that they help reinforce the notion that the bedroom should serve as a stimulus for a specific response: one not of arousal, naturally, but of sleep.

Maintain A Regular Sleep-Wake Schedule

When I see patients with sleeping problems, I often remark— only half kiddingly—that they should carve this commandment in granite and attach it to their bedroom doors:

> For your mind and body's sake,
> Each day at the same time wake.
> Once you've opened up your eyes,
> Linger not, but quickly rise.

Waking at the same hour, seven days a week, and hopping out of bed immediately will probably do more to get your sleeping pattern back on track than any other single step you can take. By now you may have guessed that establishing a constant time of waking—and, depending on the time of year, literally greeting the morning sun—serves to entrain your circadian rhythms by resetting and synchronizing your twenty-four-hour clock. It then stands to reason that if your waking rhythms are in good working order, your sleep mechanisms as well will eventually fall into step. Once these two processes are functioning smoothly, and barring any other medical or environmental disruptions, you are virtually guaranteed a good night's sleep. As we've seen, if you awaken but linger in bed, you may fall victim to random napping, with subsequent circadian disruption. Going to bed at the same hour each night, while to a degree less critical, is also helpful, for obvious reasons. By disciplining yourself to sleep at predictable times, you make your body's efforts to maintain proper circadian rhythms just that much easier.

At Night, Sleep Only When Sleepy

There's an almost Zen-like elegance to this rule. The point is this: once you've established a steady sleep-wake schedule, it is better on occasion to stay awake another hour or so than to lie in bed unable to sleep—a situation one perceptive writer in ancient Egypt aptly described as a "living hell." The basis for this principle, again, involves circadian rhythmicity. Some research suggests that there may be a window of time, probably no more than ten or fifteen minutes out of a basic ninety-minute cycle, during which the possibility of sleep reaches its optimal level. If you don't happen to be in bed during that interval, it is possible that sleep will not come until the next window arrives, an hour or so hence. According to this theory, it is counterproductive to lie in bed waiting for sleep to come. Better to rise and engage in some tranquil activity, such as one of those I'll describe in a moment, than to engage in a losing effort to force yourself to sleep.

Use the Bed for Sleep

I mentioned this earlier, but I want to reiterate the point here. Once in bed, sleep (or make love, then sleep). Don't eat, don't chat on the phone, don't watch TV. Don't discuss family finances; don't argue with your partner. And don't let the stresses and emotional upsets of the day insinuate themselves into the bed like cracker crumbs. Bed should be a stimulus that prompts one response and one response only: sleep.

Sex, as noted, is the exception to this rule. Interestingly, the male is more likely to fall asleep after intercourse than the female. What's more, the stages of sleep in men are largely the same after coitus as on other nights. Conversely, following intercourse women experience less deep sleep and more light NREM and REM sleep than on nights without sexual activity. One theory that may account for these differences is that women are statistically less likely to experience orgasm and the subsequent release of tension and feelings of relaxation. In fact, 60 to 70 percent of women who complain of insomnia also report high degrees of sexual frustration. If you feel that sexual dissatisfaction may be contributing to your inability to enjoy good sleep, discuss the matter with your partner. A little experimenting or inventiveness may help alleviate the problem. If your case is more serious, you should seek the advice of a qualified marital counselor or sex therapist. Of course, a satisfactory sex life can help make your days, as well as your nights, more fulfilling.

Establish Bedtime Rituals

These rituals, enjoyed during the half-hour or so before you hit the sack, can be anything that helps you relax as you prepare to turn in. A bath or shower can make you feel clean and calm. Careful, though: water that is too hot or too cold can be counterproductive, causing sleep-disrupting changes in your body temperature. Warm or tepid water will help you feel cool and relaxed; a cool compress placed on your eyes and forehead can also be soothing. Some people have a ritual of going around the house checking all the windows and doors to be sure they are locked; others thoughtfully select the clothes they will wear in the morning. Some people assume specific postures as they climb into bed; others indulge in a certain fantasy (not necessarily sexual in nature). One patient told me he couldn't sleep unless he had tapped quietly on the bedpost with his wedding ring— exactly four times, once for each member of his family.

To Sleep Heavily, Eat Lightly

As I've said, late meals militate against good sleep. Conversely, hunger can disturb sleep, so avoid going to bed hungry. A light snack is acceptable. And yes, warm milk or Ovaltine can be a good idea, provided you are able to digest milk properly. Be advised, however, that drinking even one glass of liquid at bedtime may prompt a sleep-disrupting trip to the bathroom at an inconvenient hour. Earlier in this chapter I presented a list of foods thought to facilitate sleep.

Put Your Mind At Ease

If the act of going to sleep makes you feel anxious about the safety and security of yourself and your family, take active steps to help provide reassurance that all is well in your household. Make it part of your ritual to test the locks on the doors and windows. Check to be sure the oven and the burners on the stove are turned off. Leave a few strategic lights burning, or place night-lights in appropriate locations, to guide your steps should you or a family member awaken during the night. Muffle disruptive sounds, such as clanky radiators or noisy pipes. Install smoke detectors and, if necessary, an electronic burglar alarm system. It's a good idea on general principles to conduct fire and tornado drills with the members of the family in order to rehearse your reactions to emergency situations. Keep the phone numbers of the police and fire departments, as well as of your doctors, prominently displayed by every telephone in the house.

SLEEP-INDUCING STRATEGIES

Assume at this point that you have adopted appropriate changes in your daily lifestyle, and that you have created the proper bedroom environment and have practiced good sleep hygiene. What if you still find yourself lying in bed, eyes open, haunted by the fear that sleep will elude you for yet another night? What now?

Count Sheep

Corny as it may sound, counting sheep or engaging in other similar repetitious activities actually does help (unless, as one expert points out, you are a sheep rancher). Similarly, you might try plucking the petals from imaginary daisies or performing mental gymnastics. Obviously the goal is not to see how high you can count but rather to focus the mind on meaningless repetitive thought patterns, in a willful effort to prevent other, more harmful thoughts from dominating your waning consciousness.

Among the techniques sleep experts have proposed, with high measures of success, are the following.

* Count ceiling tiles; when finished, count them again.
* Count backwards from 768 by 17s.
* Write the numbers from 1 to 100 on an imaginary blackboard, erasing each one in sequence; then go backwards in similar fashion.
* Recite a poem; recite it again, spelling every word.
* Devise a category—American states, four-legged animals— and think of every appropriate entry you can.
* Notice the arrival of a random thought; when the second random thought occurs, find some logical way to connect them.

Continue to link each new thought to the previous ones as it appears. This process is known as "chunking."
* Tell yourself a story, focusing not on events but on every possible irrelevant detail: the loose threads on a man's shirt, the rhythm of a woman's walk, the number and appearance of bricks in a building.
* Focus on bodily sensations. Note the feel of the sheet against your toes; listen to the gentle whirring of the furnace in the basement below.
* Place yourself in an imaginary setting—a beach, a forest, a hilltop. Concentrate on the sights and sounds: the crashing of waves on the shore and the rattle of sand as the water recedes; the feel of the sun; the smell of the grass and trees. Walk through the setting, participating in the scene rather than standing outside and watching it.

One point I should make about these strategies is that they are designed for people who have trouble sleeping. Good sleepers, on the other hand, are likely to be kept awake if they try to solve mathematical problems or envision themselves walking along the beach.

One of the techniques of Zen meditation may help you: breathe deeply and slowly, counting each breath as you inhale. When you reach four, or five, or ten, start over again. If active thoughts begin to infiltrate, you may find it helpful to imagine the thought being written on a blackboard, then imagine it being erased before you have time to read it. The effect is to create a mind unburdened by words or logical thoughts.

One sleep lab found that providing troubled sleepers with a single musical tone that was switched on and off at intervals helped people fall asleep faster than either total silence or a single unbroken sound. The technique was even more effective if the subjects counted the tones as they dropped off to sleep. This suggests to me that a metronome, set to a slow rhythm, may have a similar effect, though I have not tested the idea on a patient.

If after fifteen to thirty minutes of lying in bed trying these mental relaxation exercises you are still awake, give up for the time being. As I mentioned, you may have missed the sleep window for that particular circadian cycle. In any case get out of bed. You'll accomplish nothing by lying awake fretting about your inability to sleep. Instead go to a different room and begin some nonchallenging, repetitive activity. Do needlepoint; hook a rug; examine the furniture; paste stamps in an album; solve an easy crossword or word-search puzzle. If you read, read a textbook or a technical manual. Don't pick up one of those books you can't put down; you'll never get back to sleep that way. Watching TV is acceptable, if you choose your fare carefully and don't watch it in the bedroom. By no means should you reward your insomnia with some pleasing activity, such as reading an engrossing magazine article or gorging on a bowl of ice cream. Doing so poses the risk of training your body to awaken in order to enjoy such pleasures. If all else fails, force yourself to read this paragraph one hundred times in a row. That should do it. After forty-five minutes or so, or whenever you start to feel sleepy, return to bed. Again, though, if you can't sleep, repeat the cycle.

Still awake? Don't despair. A number of more structured relaxation techniques are at your disposal.

Relax and Sleep

Progressive relaxation, for example, is the process by which you tense and relax various muscle groups in your body. This technique, taught to such diverse people as actors and expectant mothers, involves isolating muscles—beginning, say, with the toes and working your way up the body. Tense or flex the muscle for a count of five, then release the tension. Breathe; count to ten; flex and release again. Repeat the cycle with the foot, the ankle, the calf, and so on, until you have exercised the fingers, neck, jaws, cheeks, and forehead. Don't tense so much that you get a cramp. Concentrate on the sensations; tense only one set of muscles while keeping all others relaxed.

A variation on this technique involves *autogenic suggestion,* a fancy phrase that in translation means the process of imagining that a part of your body—your hand, for example—is growing increasingly heavy, or warm. Repeat with different parts until your entire body is as heavy as lead, or as warm as toast. Similarly, autosuggestion—a mild form of self-hypnosis—calls for you to repeat a phrase, such as "I am going to sleep," over and over again.

The theory behind the sleep-inducing power of such activities, which are technically known as *cognitive focusing,* is that the act of concentrating your attention on relatively pleasant, monotonous internal sensations is intrinsically incompatible with the thoughts and images that tend to prevent the onset of sleep. Interestingly, experts believe that the specific act of cognitive focusing, rather than the process of tension release, is the mechanism that actually brings about sleep.

Sleep Less to Sleep More?

One final sleep-inducing strategy I would like to cover is the technique of *sleep restriction,* used in cases where the insomniac tends to stay in bed for eight or nine hours but enjoys only about five or six hours of sleep. Sleep restriction involves reducing the actual time spent in bed—say, by half an hour a night over a period of a week or so. Eventually patients find that only about thirty minutes of their time in bed is spent awake; the rest of the time is effective, concentrated sleep.

Results of sleep restriction have shown that it can be an effective alternative to hypnotic drugs, use of which will be covered in detail in Chapter 11. At this point, however, I want to mention one study which indicated that simple aspirin appeared to help some insomniacs by allowing them to sleep longer and awaken less frequently than they did with a placebo. These researchers believed something in the compound of the tablet, not the actual painkiller itself, was responsible. But ask your doctor before you begin taking this or any other medication.

A WORD ABOUT THE ELDERLY

As we have seen, the elderly are particularly susceptible to sleep disturbances. Aging causes the various organs and systems to deteriorate, resulting in a host of medical problems. In the brain, to take one specific case, neurons may cease to function; the level of blood flow may drop, and plaque may accumulate in the blood vessels. And when one system begins to fail, it can cause disruptions in others as well. Alzheimer's dementia, for example, may cause degeneration in the area of the brain responsible for controlling breathing during sleep and thus may

contribute to a condition of sleep apnea; lower oxygen levels may
lead in turn to further mental confusion.

Often in the elderly, circadian rhythms begin to desynchro-
nize. Thus Alzheimer's may further contribute to insomnia by
resetting the brain's biological clock. Changes in the sleep
cycle—loss of deep slow-wave sleep, for example—also reduce
the quality of sleep. Predictably, as people age they are more
prone to the effects of jet lag or other disruptions in their time
schedules, such as those resulting from the demands of shift
work.

What's more, the various medications used to treat medical
conditions can complicate matters. Add to that the various social
and environmental factors that affect sleep—reduced contact
with other people, less access to intellectual and cultural stimulation, lack of exercise—and it's not surprising that, according
to one expert, as many as 99 percent of elderly people are estimated to suffer from disturbed sleep to one degree or another.
The disruptive nighttime behavior of sleep-disturbed persons is
the main reason given by families for deciding to commit their
elderly relatives to chronic care in institutions such as nursing
homes.

As I have said, it is fallacious to assume that the elderly simply
need less sleep than younger people. A number of studies have
shown that older individuals require the same amount of sleep
they have always had; unfortunately, their bodies are less able
to provide that amount.

Identifiable sleep disorders, especially apnea, nocturnal myoclonus, and narcolepsy, account for nearly 90 percent of sleep
problems in the elderly. We have seen that simply prescribing
hypnotic drugs to bring about sleep will not help these conditions; in fact, such drugs are likely to aggravate the situation.
Proper handling of disturbed sleep in the elderly, as in any age
group, requires a careful evaluation and a multidimensional
approach to therapy. It is thus even more important for this
group to see a physician as the first step toward managing a sleep
disorder. If the patient has been taking sleeping medications for
some time, it may be necessary to begin the process of weaning
from the drug in order to ease the return to a more self-regulated
sleep pattern.

As I have noted, such major life events as retirement can

produce transient insomnia. In these cases behavior modification therapy may provide some benefits. If necessary, low doses of benzodiazepine drugs may also help for a short time, provided there exists no medical condition that would preclude their use. Those drugs with short half-lives are better; the lowered metabolism rates of the elderly reduce their ability to clear the longer-acting drugs from the system and may produce symptoms of excessive daytime sleepiness, not to mention other toxic effects.

Many of the sleep hygiene principles outlined in this chapter apply to the management of insomnia problems in older individuals as well. For example, maintaining regular sleep and rising times can do much to help structure healthier sleep patterns. Of course, the bedroom environment should be made comfortable. Some people prefer to keep the thermostat set higher than in their younger years, perhaps because differences in blood circulation make them more susceptible to cold. Caffeine should be avoided, especially from about four o'clock on; some experts even urge no caffeine after midday. One possible exception to the rules: a study of geriatric patients found that a judicious glass of wine in the evening resulted in a major drop in the use of the sedative-hypnotic drug chloral hydrate.

Some gerontologists particularly recommend adopting long and soothing rituals as a prelude to sleep. Soaking in a tub, enjoying a back massage, or sexual activity, including masturbation, can be relaxing at any stage of life. Maintaining a reasonably firm schedule during the day—rising at set times, eating regular meals, planning chores or outings at certain periods—helps establish circadian cycles. As with others, naps should be reduced or eliminated entirely, and bedtime should not come too early. Hobbies or social activities can fill the hours pleasantly and satisfyingly.

One vital principle is to make sure that an elderly person who experiences an occasional sleepless night realizes that worrying about insomnia will only worsen the situation. If the individual wakes and is unable to return to sleep, simply getting out of bed and engaging in some pleasant and relaxing activity, such as reading a book or writing a letter, will do a great deal to facilitate the return of sleepiness.

9

Help Your Child Get a Good Night's Sleep

In my discussion of parasomnias I described the types of sleep-disturbing events that primarily affect children and indicated some of the management techniques available to help minimize those problems. At this point I would like to offer some additional suggestions for improving the sleep hygiene of children.

As every parent knows, getting children into bed and keeping them there long enough to enjoy a decent night's sleep is a form of power struggle—one that can continue, like the siege of Troy, for ten years. However, there are many steps you can take to help make bedtime a more relaxed affair, to which the child may actually look forward. And, as with so many other sleep-improvement methods, success comes only with commitment and dedication to the plan.

SLEEP WITHOUT TEARS

Crying, especially in infants, is perhaps the most distressing element parents must contend with while putting the child to bed or, even worse, in the middle of the night. The reasons for crying vary, of course, but among the more likely causes are

* physical discomfort (wet diaper, room temperature too warm or too cool, inadequate or uncomfortable sleepwear, entangled bedclothes)
* hunger or thirst
* illness (ear infection, for example)
* teething
* growth spurts, especially around the ages of six months and one year
* dreams or night terrors
* an upset in the daily routine
* too much stimulation, especially right at bedtime
* fear of darkness
* fear of separation
* tension or anxiety in the home

In cases where crying has some immediately recognizable cause—hunger, for example—the remedy should be obvious. Similarly, the symptoms of illness or teething are sometimes easily relieved by administering the appropriate medication, such as nonaspirin pain relievers or children's cold formulas—of course, always following the advice of your pediatrician. Night terrors are covered in Chapter 12.

The other causes of bedtime crying are more subtle, having their roots in daytime activities and parental attitudes; the methods for bringing relief are thus more demanding. For example, children thrive on routine. Knowing that one event always follows another in a certain pattern provides reassurance that things are predictable and under control and reduces the anxiety children may have about their environment. When that routine is upset—during a holiday or vacation, for example, or by a sudden trip to Grandma's or a visit by the baby-sitter—things suddenly become different. The rules, the players, even the playing field, have changed, sometimes without warning. Not knowing what to expect or how to react, the child is liable to feel anxiety. In that case the process of going to bed only adds to the upset, with crying the likely result. A change in routine is not always so pronounced; sometimes just eating dinner an hour later, or giving the bath before dinner instead of the other way around, can create confusion and frustrate a child's expectations.

Similarly, overstimulation during the day can make it difficult for a child to wind down enough to go to bed calmly. Sometimes the stimulation comes from a houseful of visiting relatives, all of whom are trying to engage the child in play. A trip to the mall, with its sights, sounds, and crowds, can set anyone's nerves on edge, let alone a vulnerable child's. And a parent's well-intentioned efforts to prepare the child for tomorrow's event—"Guess where we're going tomorrow—to the zoo!"—can fire a young imagination to the point of disrupting sleep. Sometimes, too, seemingly harmless play activities can militate against sleep. Marching around the house banging on a drum and blowing a horn in a prebedtime parade or even simply watching inappropriate television programs or videotapes can delay the onset of sleep.

Naturally, fear of darkness or of being separated from parents can cause the bedtime ritual to become a time of terror, to the point where the mere mention of the word "bed" can trigger a tantrum. A child susceptible to such fears is also at risk of developing a conditioned response in which waking causes agitation, which in turn causes more waking and thus more agitation. In a very short time such a pattern can become a habit.

In addition to these factors, a number of environmental disturbances can harm sleep. As you are no doubt aware, children are particularly sensitive to stress and tension in the atmosphere of the home; they are uncannily adept at picking up signals of anxiety or disharmony between parents. Unable to react verbally or to cope emotionally with the fear such discord can instill, the child is likely to react in indirect ways, such as disturbed appetite or sleep. What's more, the very effort of raising a small child—including, no doubt, the inevitable loss of sleep suffered especially by the mother—further contributes to the strain in the atmosphere. In some cases poor or inadequate housing may necessitate having two or three children sleep in the same room as the parents. Obviously, crying by one child in such circumstances destroys the sleep not only of the child but of siblings and parents as well. Tragically, lack of sleep is often cited as a contributing factor in instances of child abuse.

There are many different schools of thought on managing crying. An entire generation of children was raised on the Dr. Spock method, which encourages parents to allow the child to cry for a period of time over the course of a few nights. The theory holds, and many parents find it true, that the first night is the most difficult, as the child is likely to cry for a half-hour or more. On the second night the crying period should diminish to about ten minutes; on subsequent nights it should eventually vanish altogether. The principle is that the child finally learns that bedtime crying brings no response, or at most a limited response, from parents and is thus literally a waste of breath. The technique is particularly effective if the child has been a good sleeper in the past but has suffered a recent disruption in sleep pattern due to illness or some other cause.

Other experts, however, believe that telling parents to ignore crying goes against their natural instincts to comfort and soothe the child. They make the point that a child who feels its cries are ignored may turn its emotions inward, which may cause complications at later stages of life.

Still others advocate a more balanced approach, treading a fine line between ignoring the crying and reacting to it immediately every time. In this strategy, the parents are permitted to rock the child to sleep in the crib. Later, they are to stop rocking, but may keep a hand placed lightly on the child's back. Then they may sit in the room but without touching the child. A few days later they will sit outside the room with the door open. Finally they will put the child gently to bed and leave the area entirely. The plan is not foolproof; there may still be occasional crying. Parents are permitted to respond in an appropriate controlled fashion: entering the room and speaking reassuringly, for example, but not picking the child up or rocking until sleep returns.

SLEEP STRATEGIES FOR CHILDREN

Decisions on how to cope with child-raising issues are highly personal and sensitive matters; I would not presume to issue sweeping general edicts on how to handle your particular situation. The choice is yours. However, there are a number of other recognized strategies, appropriate to growth and development,

which you may wish to try in order to help forestall sleep problems, and which may actually bring about improvements in your
child's sleeping patterns. In many cases, these approaches require the collaboration and mutual support of both parents.

Maintain a Positive Emotional Atmosphere in the Home

Remember that your anxiety will become your child's anxiety.
Thoroughly examine your relationship with your spouse and
with your children to see if there are deep-seated problems. If
you experience more than the usual stress, you may do everyone
in your family a favor if you seek professional help.

Arrange Living Space to Facilitate Sleep

Obviously, most people can't just run out and buy a larger
house. But there may be less drastic steps you can take—building interior walls, reassigning use of living space—that will help
everyone breathe (and sleep) easier.

Establish a Bedtime Ritual

Devise a series of four or five activities that serve to prepare
the child for bed in a progressively quiet and calming fashion.
For example, you may wish to allow the child to burn off excess
energy by roughhousing and romping shortly after dinner. Similarly, if bathtime is a time of splashing and frantic fun, give the
bath at least an hour or two before sleep, so that the hilarity has
some time to wear off. Then take the steps necessary to ready the
child for bed—dressing, having a snack, brushing teeth—so that
when sleep comes you don't have to interrupt the process by
scrambling to stuff him or her into sleepwear. If appropriate, you
might then allow the child a half-hour or so of quiet time alone,
to play with toys or explore the bedroom. At that point a few
quiet songs or lap games may be in order, followed by a soothing
story or two. Many parents find that using a specific and final
farewell, in the form of a certain poem or gesture—such as a

prayer or a kiss on the nose—helps make the point that the ritual has ended and the time for sleep has come.

Minimize Disruptions in Your Routine

Naturally we all look forward to special events such as visits with friends or relatives, family outings, or even such simple pleasures as a meal at a new restaurant. As we have discussed, however, such activities can take their toll. The more you can anticipate a forthcoming change in schedule, the better prepared you'll be to cope with your child's disrupted sleep the following night. Plan the activity to coincide as much as possible with your child's routine of eating and nap taking. Bring along favorite toys or books to create an environment populated by familiar things. Conduct your usual sleep ritual—bathtime, stories, and so on—to the degree possible in the new situation.

Discover—and Respect—Your Child's Sleep Rhythms

As I have emphasized, a constant time of rising is a key element in structuring sleep. The same principle applies to children. By waking children at the same time every morning, you help them set their circadian clocks. You will soon notice the point in the evening at which they begin to grow sleepy, and can then begin to establish a sleep routine that reflects their needs without forcing them to conform to an arbitrary and unworkable schedule.

Establish a Bedtime Time Cue

Associate bedtime with a neutral—and implacable—time cue, such as the position of the hands on a clock, the ringing of a kitchen timer, or the conclusion of a certain television program. By doing so, you assign the responsibility of determining bedtime to a force seemingly beyond your control or anyone else's. A child who knows the clock has reached a certain position, or who hears a bell ring, is more likely to accept the fact that bedtime, unquestionably, has arrived.

Don't Force a Child to Sleep

Remember that bedtime and sleeptime are not synonymous. You might put the child in bed at eight o'clock, for example, but you should allow a half-hour or so for quiet activity—playing with favorite stuffed animals or looking at treasured picture books. After a reasonable winding-down period, firmly but gently insist that lights go out and activity stop for the night.

Don't Isolate the Child

The bedroom environment of a child, like that of an adult, should be conducive to sleep, not frightening. By all means use a night-light, if necessary. In some cases even a low-wattage lamp can help, rather than hinder, sleep. Keep the door open, or ajar, so children know that they have access to you, or that you will hear them, in case they need you. Some parents have found that playing a tape of children's songs or their own voices, or leaving a radio tuned to a classical music station, facilitates sleep and provides a reassuring presence in the room.

Help the Child Rise and Shine

In the morning avoid letting the child linger in bed, dozing in intermittent intervals. Cheerfully and gently encourage the child to awaken. Raise the shades, let him or her see the new morning, and describe the events of the day ahead.

As I mentioned earlier, many cultures feel that allowing the child to sleep in the parents' bed helps forestall, or minimize, the problems of nighttime wakings. Some experts encourage the use of a "family bed"; many parents are actually relieved to know that such an option may be a reasonable solution in their case. Others are concerned that this approach only postpones children's inevitable separation from their parents. Such a decision is entirely up to you. You may wish to discuss the question with other parents in your community or seek the guidance of a children's psychologist or parents' support group.

Other steps you might take depend on the child's age and abilities. Sometimes altering the timing and duration of naps can help a young child sleep more soundly at night. With an infant about six months or older you may find that offering a nighttime meal of rice cereal or farina improves sleep. Many authorities believe that gradually tapering off feedings in the early hours of sleep helps a child learn to sleep through the night. The idea is that a child whose last waking memory is of a breast or a bottle will awaken with the desire to have that stimulus restored. In contrast, others believe that a child who is being breast-fed should be given meals on demand.

Be Firm with Your Child

In children aged ten years or older, most chronic sleep problems are behavioral in origin and are usually related to a well-meaning but misguided effort by the parents to manage a temporary sleep disturbance. The challenge is to show proper concern for the child's sleep disruption during an awakening while avoiding the tendency to reinforce or inadvertently reward the behavior that led to the problem in the first place. If children are old enough, discuss the situation with them. Let them know you are sensitive to and concerned about their problem, whether it is nighttime awakenings or bed-wetting. Sometimes just knowing that parents care enough to try to understand can effect a cure. If corrective steps are taken, institute them firmly and consistently. For example, if your child tends to wander, unwelcome, into your bed at night, it may be necessary to lock the bedroom door (after first carefully explaining the reason for doing so). You may have to put up with strong protest, but by standing your ground, and reinforcing proper behavior with praise and other rewards (such as special treats or activities), you will soon see a change in your child's pattern.

If the source of your child's sleep disruption is medical in origin, rather than emotional or behavioral, appropriate therapy is of course called for. For example, children with sleep apnea, usually detected by its symptom of excessive daytime sleepiness, should be assessed by a physician to determine if some structural abnormality of the throat is contributing to the problem. In such cases it may be helpful to record your child's snores and supply the tape to the doctor for analysis.

I am extremely reluctant to prescribe drugs for children with sleep problems. In severe cases some physicians may recommend the use of the hypnotic drugs phenergan or chloral hydrate, but usually such a step is called for only if some occurrence such as illness or hospitalization has disrupted the child's sleep pattern. As with any drugs there are risks, not the least of which is a potential worsening of the child's ability to sleep. I am much more inclined to urge behavioral or other methods to help correct a temporary sleep disruption in a child.

I want to mention, too, that there is a British physician whose prescription for sleep disturbance is an overnight stay in the hospital. He reports that such a drastic step, usually reserved for single-parent families, works in difficult cases for several reasons: it dramatizes to parent and child alike the seriousness of the situation; it breaks the usual sleep pattern by removing the child from the source of difficulty—and it gives the single mother or father a much-needed respite from her or his demanding child.

10

Professional Solutions

If you have made a conscientious effort to improve your bedtime habits and hygiene yet find yourself still unable to get a decent night's rest or stay alert during the day, it may be time to seek professional advice. While it is true that sleep disorders represent a relatively new field of medicine, it is also true that the ability of physicians to identify and treat the causes of insomnia continues to grow. And for particularly difficult cases, the advent of sleep-disorders centers—clinical laboratories devoted to the detection of sleep problems—has created the opportunity to study the process of sleep in a way never before possible. Armed with precise and comprehensive data generated by a sleep lab, physicians can determine the course of therapy most likely to produce the best results.

What is your first step in seeking medical help? The answer depends on a number of factors, but the best option is probably the one closest at hand: see your family doctor. When the patient is a child, a pediatrician should be consulted. If you have been seeing a particular doctor more or less regularly over the years, he or she will of course be familiar with your medical history and your general state of health. The records on file may contain clues about the origin of your sleep problem or may shed some light on any current disruptions in your well-being. And like many people, you may even have come to consider your family physician or general practitioner a trusted friend and ally. If you don't know a doctor in your community, ask a friend to recommend one, or call your state or local medical society for a referral.

However, keep in mind that the degree of success you have with this physician—or with any doctor—depends in large measure on the honesty and thoroughness with which you present the details of your complaint. You may feel reluctant, for example, to reveal to this friend of the family the fact that you have a habit of drinking two or three cocktails after dinner or that you still smoke a pack of cigarettes a day despite your repeated pledges to quit. Such reticence, while perfectly understandable, can thwart the healing process before it has even begun. Therefore, if you feel you are unable to confide in your regular doctor, you may be better off seeking help from another physician or professional.

Family physicians and general practitioners as a rule possess many of the skills needed to cope with insomnia-related conditions, including basic psychiatric techniques. Pediatricians are particularly skilled at dealing with parasomnias in children. But having said that, I must reiterate that sleep disturbance is a multifaceted and notoriously difficult problem to dissect and analyze. And, as in any profession, abilities can vary. Some doctors, on hearing the word "insomnia," instinctively reach for their pens, scribble a prescription for a hypnotic drug, and consider the matter closed. We have seen, however, that drugs are at best a temporary solution, a point I'll expand on later in this chapter. If you sense that your physician has not considered all aspects of your sleep disturbance or is merely taking the therapeutic path of least resistance, you would be wise to seek a second opinion. An internist, for example, may be more likely to recognize sleep problems that have arisen as a consequence of some medical illness.

Depending on the diagnosis, a sleep specialist may need to be brought in to handle difficult or intractable cases. For example, if sleep apnea is involved, a specialist trained in pulmonological disorders may be able to recommend an effective solution. Other sleep experts possess facility in such diverse areas as cardiology, endocrinology, or neurology and thus can manage conditions related to the heart, metabolism, or brain, respectively. A specialist, by definition, is trained to focus on a particular area of concern. Thus while neurologists will be able to recognize and manage a case of narcolepsy, a cardiologist is needed to handle a situation involving, say, heart failure.

If a medical diagnosis is made and confirmed, then of course the treatment will focus on correcting the specific problem. For example, if you suffer from obstructive sleep apnea, you will be asked to consider the options discussed previously, which range from surgical correction to the use of a breathing mask. Similarly, the use of diuretics may help alleviate the fluid buildup arising from congestive heart failure, while analgesics can bring relief from the chronic pain that may be disturbing your sleep.

A psychiatrist should be considered if response to the initial therapeutic approach has been unsatisfactory, or if the insomnia has been found to stem from some form of mental (as opposed to medical) abnormality. Also, if the patient is an adult and experiences a parasomnia—bed-wetting or sleepwalking, for example—then a psychiatric strategy is indicated. In dealing with sleep disorders, psychiatrists can make important and unique contributions. They are trained to treat the entire spectrum of sleep problems, medical as well as mental in origin, and to handle the psychological dimensions of insomnia as well. Some of the proven behavioral approaches to therapy, such as biofeedback, are best managed by psychiatric specialists. I'll describe some of the various psychotherapeutic options shortly.

Regardless of your point of entry into the healthcare system, the management of your insomnia, as I've stressed repeatedly, is multidimensional in nature. Personal improvements in sleep habits and lifestyle, working in combination with medical therapies—behavioral, psychological, pharmaceutical—offer the greatest hope for improvement in your sleep during the night and your ability to function during the day.

The consensus among experts is that the first step, following a thorough medical evaluation, is to improve sleep hygiene, particularly by withdrawal from alcohol and unnecessary drugs, including sleep medications. Attention is then focused on implementing such practices as maintaining regular sleep and rising times. Behavioral or relaxation therapy may also be appropriate. (Not all insomniacs are mentally or physically tense, however; for such people relaxation techniques may be counterproductive.)

The temporary use of certain drugs for sleep may help break the pattern of insomnia symptoms, at least to the point where other, more effective, long-term therapies may begin. In cases where situational or psychological issues are major factors, a psychiatric evaluation is crucial. Depending on the nature of these issues, various techniques may prove useful, including stress reduction and supportive therapy or other psychotherapy to improve self-image or interpersonal relationships. Education and reassurance are essential elements, regardless of the psychotherapeutic strategy. Use of drugs at this point should be targeted to a psychiatric condition, such as endogenous depression. If after these steps the insomnia persists, a visit to a sleep lab is indicated to provide the missing information needed to solve the problem.

Let's look now at each of these stages of management in more detail.

PSYCHOTHERAPEUTIC AND BEHAVIORAL APPROACHES

Before psychiatric therapy can be effective, the use of drugs and alcohol must be diminished gradually. Sometimes education and reassurance are all that's needed; other, more serious drug and alcohol problems may require specialized help. Some insomniacs become dependent on their nightly drink or sleeping pill and may tend to panic without it, obviously making the withdrawal process more difficult. The goal should be to begin with as clean a slate as possible, so that more appropriate and effective therapies can be allowed to work. If you cannot control your alcohol or drug consumption, ask your psychiatrist or therapist to recommend a specialist.

Attention is then turned to managing the emotional and stress factors causing the mental and physiological turmoil that lies at the root of most insomnias. With psychotherapy, patients gain insight into the direct connection between stress and sleeplessness, or learn how to recognize and express anger or conflict in appropriate ways. They are encouraged to accept and tolerate occasional periods of sleeplessness; in so doing they break the vicious circle whereby fear about their inability to sleep ironically results in, or aggravates, insomnia. Certain physical strategies help the body relax, while mental strategies help transform harmful thought patterns, such as nighttime rumination or worry, into beneficial ones which induce a sense of calm, reassurance, and tranquillity. When a psychiatric illness is present, such as depression or personality disorder, appropriate measures will of course result not only in an improved ability to sleep but in a better overall sense of wellbeing. As befits the complex nature of insomnia, a psychotherapeutic strategy that combines supportive, insight-oriented, and behavioral approaches has the greatest chance of succeeding.

I must point out that the process of psychotherapy can be a difficult one, made even more difficult by some of the very personality traits that cause insomnia in the first place. For example, poor sleepers who dwell exclusively on the symptom of sleeplessness may be extremely reluctant to explore the psychological cause of their problem. They may insist that all they need is a sleeping pill, when what they really need is to look deeply at their emotional responses to the process of going to sleep, to learn whether some long-buried fear is disrupting their physiological sleep mechanisms. A psychotherapeutic approach that is analytical in nature can help uncover these deeply buried feelings.

There are other issues as well: patients may deny that a problem exists; they may resist the doctor's advice or otherwise struggle for control. Conversely, some patients become so dependent on their doctors that they are unable to break away and manage their situations independent of medical guidance. I mention this not to bewail the professional problems I encounter in my psychiatric practice but to stress that if you undertake therapy you should do so with commitment and dedication to the plan—not because it makes the psychiatrist's job easier (although it does) but because it is the only attitude that can improve the chances for a successful outcome.

There is no doubt that psychotherapy can help relieve insomnia. One study of over 25,000 patients found that those who received some form of psychotherapy experienced more improvement in their symptoms, and in their overall sense of functioning, than 85 percent of those who did not receive therapy. In addition to its high degree of effectiveness, psychotherapy has been shown to cost less than other forms of medical treatment, in part because it reduces the patient's need to rely on drugs.

The actual course of psychotherapy your physician recommends may depend on the nature of your insomnia and on your emotional and environmental circumstances. In cases of transient insomnia—short-lived sleeplessness caused by sudden disruptions in the pattern of living—supportive therapy is usually all that's needed.

Supportive Psychotherapy and Insight-oriented Therapy

Supportive therapy, as its name implies, focuses on helping patients recognize the cause of their problem and reassuring them that the insomnia is only temporary and that their previous ability to function will return. Through education patients learn about the sleep process and how to master the life stresses that can disrupt it, and to do so before the pattern of sleeplessness becomes entrenched as a form of learned negative behavior. Supportive therapy helps patients to conquer the fear of sleeplessness and encourages them to discharge emotional arousal by promoting exercise, analyzing anger-provoking incidents, and using such classic therapeutic techniques as role-playing.

Also appropriate for transient insomnia is insight-oriented therapy, whose goal is to help the patient penetrate and discover the root fear or psychological cause of the insomnia. A combination of insight-oriented and supportive therapy is likely to be more effective than either approach alone. Because transient insomnia by definition passes quickly (within three weeks or less), supportive and insight-oriented therapies are similarly short-term.

Psychodynamic Therapy for Chronic Insomnia

Somewhat more complicated, of course, are cases of chronic insomnia. A long-term insomniac is more likely to deny that a psychological problem exists and thus will be more resistant to treatment. What's more, as we have seen, there is a danger of "secondary gains" whereby patients actually come to enjoy the effects of their illness: sympathy from concerned relatives, attention from doctors, reduced levels of responsibility within the home, on the job, and in society. And the longer the insomnia persists, the more self-perpetuating it becomes. The tasks of psychotherapy, then, become somewhat more complex, as the physician must not only remedy the disorder but also overcome the problems of resistance and denial.

Judicious use of drugs is sometimes called for in the initial stages of treatment of chronic insomnia. Short courses of therapy with benzodiazepines can produce quick relief of symptoms and help break the pattern of sleeplessness, allowing the patient to begin focusing on other psychotherapeutic strategies. The drug must be chosen with regard for a number of factors involved in the patient's individual case. As a rule it should be discontinued after a few days, or a few weeks at most, so that long-term solutions can be brought to bear.

Supportive therapy plays the same important role in managing chronic insomnia as it does in transient insomnia. But other strategies must also come into play. One of these is psychodynamic therapy, a term whose roots translate roughly as "movement of the mind." The name is appropriate, because under psychodynamic therapy patients gain insight into unexpressed psychic conflicts and feelings—for example, feelings of aggression—which have been buried deep within. In so doing patients experience a revolution in their manner of thought and, subsequently, behavior.

Psychodynamic therapy seeks to clarify the specific issues that may be triggering the insomnia, then encourages the patient to interpret the problem so that it may be confronted and so that he or she can begin to work toward a solution. Emphasis is placed not only on the immediate problem of sleeplessness but on the underlying causes as well. For such an approach to succeed the patient must be willing and able to communicate effectively with the therapist in order to participate actively in the healing process. In addition, he or she must be highly motivated and possess a certain measure of intelligence. By intelligence I don't mean book learning; intelligence in this sense simply means the ability to think in ways appropriate to the task at hand. If the patient is unwilling to explore the unpleasant memories of childhood or is mentally impaired, for example, some other therapeutic strategy is called for.

Interpersonal Therapy for Chronic Insomnia

Depending on the individual circumstances, the patient may also benefit from an approach that incorporates interpersonal therapy—therapy that focuses on relationships with other people. This can take any number of forms.

Group therapy, as you are probably aware, involves discussions and structured encounters among a number of people. The advantages of such a technique are many. The patient is given a chance to express feelings to a group of people who are predisposed to understand the nature of the problem. In addition, the patient hears from others in similar circumstances and can compare and contrast experiences. In many instances the reactions and suggestions of peers can have much more dramatic impact than advice given by a paid professional. Alcoholics Anonymous is considered to be a form of interpersonal or group therapy.

Marital counseling or sexual counseling may be indicated in situations where the primary cause of sleep difficulty is perceived to be sexual or to involve a spouse or partner. One complaint I often hear is that patients with insomnia are "too tired" to participate in sexual relations. Counseling can uncover the motivations that lie behind such behavior. These discoveries help patients realize the unconscious control they exercise over their mates by exploiting their chronic fatigue in such a way, and can help the couple return to a more satisfying level of marital or sexual relationship.

Behavioral Therapy

The therapies discussed so far are focused on reorienting the emotional reactions to stress in order to cope with the problem of sleeplessness. Another major therapeutic category is that of *behavioral therapy,* the goal of which is to bring about changes in habits and other physiological functioning. Such an approach concentrates on the use of relaxation techniques and other structured modifications in the ways patients think or behave. As a rule behavioral therapy—considered to be most effective if the insomnia problem is one of falling asleep—is used in conjunction with one of the forms of psychological therapy described above, because it deals primarily with the symptoms, not the causes, of the problem. This is especially true when the insomnia arises as a result of some other condition such as depression or myoclonus (night twitching). One reason behavioral therapy is effective is that patients actively and physically participate in the process and consequently can detect and monitor progress, usually within a very short time. When that happens, they begin to feel a sense of mastery over their situation—which is precisely the message the psychiatrist dealing with insomnia wishes to convey. A typical course of behavioral therapy may take about eight to ten weeks; studies indicate that as many as three out of four insomniacs respond positively to such nonpharmacological strategies.

Often the process of behavior modification can begin in the primary care setting—that is, under the guidance of a family physician or other nonpsychiatric professional. Following the medical exam the doctor will conduct an analysis of the problem, one which draws on all available sources of information including focused discussions with the patient and perhaps with relatives and friends as well. Then, depending on the nature of the problem and on the physician's own propensities, any of a number of options may be explored. Some of these, such as progressive relaxation, autogenic suggestion, and meditative techniques, were touched on in a previous chapter. In all cases the goal is to have the patient learn a relatively simple method for lowering the state of physiological arousal and inducing a feeling of calmness. Be advised, however: the effectiveness of this therapy, like any other, depends on the skill and expertise of those administering it. If you feel your counselor is not addressing your specific needs, look elsewhere.

These relaxation techniques are practiced not just at bedtime; they can and should be used two, three, or more times during the day to improve not only the ability to sleep but also the level of daytime functioning. One further point: It's best to learn and practice these techniques in some setting other than the bedroom—in a classroom or a doctor's office, for example. Doing so lowers the risk of turning the therapy itself into a stimulus that arouses you just when you should be calming down. In other words, if you go to bed at 11:30 and spend the next hour or so working on your relaxation, you are defeating the very goal you are trying to achieve.

Another behavioral strategy involves *desensitization,* a process by which the patient learns to reduce the anxiety-provoking and unhappy associations of going to bed. One technique is to keep a logbook of fears or other unpleasant feelings associated with the process of going to sleep, and rank them according to the level of anxiety they provoke. The patient is then trained to recognize the thoughts and feelings associated with the event considered to be the least anxiety-provoking, and to substitute those relatively moderate feelings whenever a more stressful situation occurs.

Another example of behavior modification is *biofeedback,* the process by which information about physiological processes and conditions is relayed to the patient, who is then encouraged to control the function and thus reduce stress. For example, an electrode placed on the fingertip can be set to trigger a tone whenever there is a drop in body temperature as small as one hundredth of a degree. By learning to relax and control vasodilation to a certain extent, the patient may be able to lower body temperature significantly and thus may facilitate the onset of sleep. Other biofeedback techniques attempt to reduce muscle tension or to produce brain waves at 14 to 16 cycles per second (the wavelength associated with the onset of sleep during Stage 1). Use of biofeedback requires the presence of a trained supervisor, as well as a considerable investment of time, equipment, and money. Insomniacs typically need between sixteen and forty sessions of biofeedback to see some improvement.

Hypnosis may work for some, but it is generally inappropriate for insomnia. The trance induced by hypnosis is not the same as sleep. It can also be awkward to call in a hypnotist whenever you are ready to turn in for the night.

Many of the self-help techniques discussed in the previous chapter are examples of the behavioral technique known as *stimulus control*—that is, they are designed to reinforce the concept that beds and bedrooms are for sleeping. As I've discussed, using the bed as a social center or work station can prevent the onset of sleep. By following certain rules—going to bed when sleepy, getting up at the same time every morning, avoiding naps—the patient is gradually trained to experience one response, and only one, upon making contact with the bed. That response, of course, is sleep.

Source attribution, a psychological method whose efficacy has not yet been clearly demonstrated in the treatment of insomnia, is the technique whereby the patient learns to redefine the source of sleeplessness as being some external or environmental factor rather than an internal emotional or mental upheaval. The theory is that when insomnia is attributed to an outside force, the problem can be more easily controlled. Usually the attribution has to do with the use of placebo medication, as described below. To use an extremely simple example of another kind, if the patient can come to believe that insomnia is caused by the ticking of an annoying clock down the hall, then by simply disposing of the clock the insomnia may be brought under control. As I said, however, not enough is known about this approach to recommend its use in insomnia.

A variation known as *control attribution* is more likely to work, especially if the insomnia is of mild to moderate severity. Under control attribution patients are taught that they are in control of the sleep process. The effect of this approach is seen in patients who are given a sleeping pill, then told later that the pill was only a placebo. Studies have found that most of these patients continue to sleep well without medication, having been led to believe that they control their own ability to sleep. It sounds sneaky, I admit, but if it works, who can argue? In any case attribution is designed to correct misconceptions about the sleep process.

The final type of behavioral therapy I want to mention is *cognitive restructuring.* In a sense this approach is a form of desensitization involving a conscious effort to turn negative thoughts into positive ones. For example, the patient may have a habit of repeating over and over again a phrase such as "I know I'll never fall asleep" or "I'm going to be so tired I'll be worthless tomorrow." Using desensitization, the patient is encouraged to substitute other thoughts, perhaps "I know I can fall asleep" or "I'll be all right, even if I don't get eight hours of sleep." Techniques such as counting sheep, performing mental exercises, or imagining oneself walking through a forest, as I mentioned earlier, are also cognitive in nature. They help facilitate sleep by focusing attention on pleasant feelings or monotonous thoughts. The basic theory is that a mind filled with beautiful or boring images has no room for troubling ones. It is possible, however, that such techniques are of somewhat more transient value and are less likely to result in deep-seated, if not permanent, changes in the patient's thought processes.

PSYCHOTHERAPY FOR MENTAL DISTURBANCES

Of course, any psychological therapy must be designed with care to address the specific problems and symptoms involved. For example, the goals in managing affective disorders such as depression differ from the goals in treating anxiety or personality disorders. As with any medical treatment, the more accurate the diagnosis, the easier it is to choose effective therapy. To achieve an accurate diagnosis, as I have so often stressed, the first steps should involve a thorough physical and a detailed patient and family history. These initial steps may indicate a physical cause (which may respond very well to treatment) for the depression or other disorder, or help diagnose the specific type of psychosis the patient may be suffering from. When treatment is concentrated on the underlying condition, either physical or psychological, the symptom we are concerned with here, insomnia, will in most cases disappear.

Depression

In depression, therapy concentrates on providing patients with a more realistic perspective on themselves and the world around them by modifying their extremely negative self-image and helping to identify, and eradicate, self-defeating behavior. Cognitive therapies, such as those described above, can help to mitigate the habit of pessimistic thinking with a more optimistic outlook. Obviously, however, merely reciting "Every day in every way I'm getting better and better" will not cure depression. Interpersonal psychotherapy often helps shore up sagging social skills or helps the patient to cope with difficulties in personal relationships. Family therapy is especially useful in identifying the problems stemming from relationships between parents and siblings, and can help patients learn to express feelings and discharge emotional tensions in ways that prevent further damage and that may actually lead to constructive results at the same time. If indicated, marital therapy can work in the same way. A combination of individual therapy and some form of interpersonal therapy provides a well-rounded approach that is often very effective.

In addition, medications when used properly may help tremendously in the treatment of depression, especially if they correct an underlying chemical imbalance that may be causing the depression. Furthermore, new and potentially exciting developments in antidepressive medication give hope of even more effective treatments in the near future.

And, in some cases, use of sleep deprivation—waking the patient from REM sleep—seems to help improve mood.

Anxiety Disorders

Patients with anxiety disorders usually respond best to some form of psychodynamic therapy, beginning with supportive therapy and drug management. A behavioral approach can help in cases of phobia or in obsessive-compulsive disorders. Education and reassurance are critical, as is training in ways to express feelings, which can help reduce the level of anxiety. If the physician feels the patient is able to handle it, insight-oriented therapy can help uncover the recurring themes that may underlie the patient's problem—for example, difficulty with authority figures stemming from a troubled early relationship with demanding parents. Treatment then concentrates on the management of these specific conflicts, in terms of emotional responses as well as behavioral patterns. Unlike depression, an anxiety disorder will not respond to sleep deprivation techniques; in fact, sleep deprivation increases the likelihood of a panic attack.

Patients who suffer from somatoform disorders—those in which the physical symptoms have no physiological basis but result from a psychological problem—are as a rule resistant to the formal psychotherapeutic process. Such a reaction is understandable, since these people are prone to discredit a direct cause-and-effect relationship between their psychic disturbance and their sleep disturbance. In such cases supportive therapy and drugs may help prepare the way for an eventual shift to insight-oriented therapy. The primary goal is to prevent further entrenchment in a lifestyle that revolves around insomnia and its symptoms.

Disorders of substance abuse, specifically alcoholism, require withdrawal from the offending element, followed by careful management of the predictable symptoms of withdrawal. As I mentioned, individual therapy combined with participation in supportive group therapy such as AA meetings is highly effective.

There is also a variety of personality disorders, such as compulsion or multiple personalities, which cause sleep disruption. Suffice it to say that treatment of each of these, as with any other psychiatric illness, depends on the severity of the illness, the patient's circumstances, and his or her ability to participate in the therapeutic process.

THE SLEEP LABORATORY

When you have a sore throat, a doctor can ask you to open your mouth and say "aah." But when you have a problem sleeping, the cause is not so easily detectable. It's not very likely that your physician will make a house call at midnight for the sole purpose of watching you try to sleep for eight hours.

In response to this situation an important diagnostic tool was devised: the sleep laboratory. In less than a decade the number of clinical facilities devoted to the study of sleeping people has risen from a baker's dozen to about ten times that many. Centers can be found in most American states, as well as in Canada, Italy, France, Japan, and the Soviet Union. Some of these are devoted exclusively to the intensive study of certain types of disorders, such as sleep apnea or the problems of children. In addition, hundreds more hospitals and medical centers now offer special expertise in the study, and correction, of sleep disorders.

Each year between 20,000 and 30,000 new patients visit these facilities in search of help. Data reveal that excessive daytime sleepiness is the predominant complaint, accounting for 42 percent of the cases seen. Of this group, seven out of ten are subsequently found to have either narcolepsy or severe sleep apnea. "Insomnia"—the inability to fall asleep or stay asleep—is the symptom of another 26 percent.

Due to the work of sleep labs there has been a surge in the flow of scientific data concerning the sleep process and the forces that disrupt it. In addition, patients who visit a lab receive more complete and accurate diagnoses of their condition. Knowing the cause of the problem then makes it possible to prescribe therapy that is appropriate and that has a much greater chance of bringing effective relief.

Can sleep labs really make a difference in the treatment of insomnia? Absolutely. It is believed that approximately 30 percent of patients with insomnia have some underlying organic disorder that would not be revealed either by an examination in a doctor's office or by a psychiatric evaluation. Thus for three out of every ten insomniacs the cause of the problem may only be discovered within a sleep lab.

A recent study reviewed the original diagnoses of insomnia in 123 patients as determined by office medical examinations and compared them with the findings that turned up later in the sleep lab. In almost half of those cases—49 percent, to be precise—the results of the laboratory study made it necessary to revise the previous diagnosis.

In fifty of these patients the lab findings added new information to the original diagnosis. For example, sixteen patients were found to experience nocturnal myoclonus, a problem not previously suspected. Another group of patients exhibited changes in sleep patterns that are associated with depression or some form of neurological disorder. Thirteen patients slept better in the lab than at home, indicating some unsuspected form of conditioned (psychophysiological) insomnia. Other new findings included sleep apnea, cardiac arrhythmias, and one disorder of the sleep-wake schedule (DSWS), in this case a delayed sleep phase.

Furthermore, this study found that in 20 percent of the patients, lab findings disagreed completely with the original clinical diagnosis. Nine patients, for example, who were originally thought to have either sleep apnea, arrhythmia, or myoclonus showed no signs of these conditions in the sleep lab. More significant, seventeen patients diagnosed as being depressed showed none of the sleep patterns typical of depression, such as onset of the REM state less than sixty-five minutes after the beginning of sleep. It should be obvious that wrong or incomplete diagnosis, left uncorrected, will lead to wrong or incomplete therapeutic strategies.

I mention these facts not to heap scorn on physicians who fail to spot the causes of insomnia, or to shake your faith in your doctor's expertise. My intention is to underscore how truly difficult it is to ferret out the true cause of sleeplessness. I also want to stress the growing value and importance of the sleep lab in helping to paint the most accurate diagnostic picture of insomnia that can be obtained.

At this point, let me describe the steps involved in the sleep lab process.

I should remind you, however, that a visit to a lab is usually the final stage in dealing with a sleep problem, not the first one. Although the purpose and function of labs is still controversial among sleep experts, it is generally accepted that the patients who are most likely to benefit from sleep analysis are those insomniacs who have failed to respond to the clinical interventions already discussed, including improvements in sleep habits and hygiene, withdrawal from pills and alcohol, psychotherapeutic or behavioral strategies, and in some cases limited use of sleep medications. As we have seen, these previous steps require some time before their beneficial effects are seen; consequently, physicians may not send patients to a lab for six months or more after the initial diagnosis.

You are a likely candidate for referral to a sleep lab if

* you have failed to respond to medication
* psychiatric or medical disorders have been specifically ruled out
* you suffer from severe or significant daytime sleepiness with no obvious cause
* you snore
* you have experienced an unexplained sleep complaint persisting for years

At the lab you may undergo another physical exam, and you will be given a battery of psychological tests to evaluate your personality and behavior patterns and to help uncover any recent life changes that may be affecting your sleep. You may also be given a neurological exam and other clinical tests to eliminate the possibility of some organic cause. The lab faculty—which may include a team of neurologists, psychologists, psychiatrists, and other specialists—will also review your medical and family history and will ask about your sleep history in some detail. The elements involved in taking your sleep history are

* defining your specific sleep problem
* assessing the clinical course of your condition
* distinguishing between other possible sleep or medical disorders
* reassessing the previous diagnosis
* evaluating your sleep and wakefulness patterns over the course of days or weeks
* questioning your bed partner and other family members
* evaluating the impact of the sleep disorder on your lifestyle

You will probably be asked to maintain a sleep diary, similar to the one outlined in Chapter 1, for a week or two. By providing a faithful record of your sleep habits and patterns, you will give the researchers vital clues about the nature of your sleep disorder. Among the types of information you will be asked to provide are

* times of retiring and arising
* variations in schedule between weekdays and weekends
* recent changes in the sleep-wake schedule
* subjective assessment of the quality of sleep: how sound is it? How restorative?
* amount of daily sleep needed to feel alert and energetic
* extent to which this amount of sleep is obtained
* use of drugs to regulate sleep and waking
* sleep habits in childhood and at other pertinent stages of life
* differences between quality of sleep in the past and at present
* attitudes toward sleep

* sleep patterns: falling asleep, staying asleep, morning awakening
* symptoms of sleeplessness seen during the day and their effect on functioning
* extent of daytime sleepiness
* status of the problem: is it constant? Changing? Worsening?
* napping habits
* evidence of snoring, gagging, leg jerks
* hygiene: use of drugs, alcohol, caffeine, especially after 6:00 P.M.
* current emotional or physical problems and their treatment
* bedroom environment

If you have been taking sleep medications, the lab, working in consultation with your own physician, will begin a process of withdrawal. Depending on the results of your tests, you may then be asked to spend a night in the lab.

The main goal of an overnight stay in a sleep lab room— essentially a cross between a hospital room and a motel—is to undergo a polysomnographic recording. As its name implies, polysomnography involves analyzing many different aspects of your sleep as you lie in bed; thus, to turn a phrase, it is a form of "lie" detection. During this process you are connected to a bank of monitors via pairs of electrodes taped to your chin, the corners of your eyes, your forehead, scalp, chest, and legs. A belt around your chest will also detect diaphragmatic movement. Sometimes a small microphone will be placed beneath your nose so that monitors in the adjacent room can detect snoring. The EEG is used to record sleep stages, as registered by changes in brain waves. Other monitors record the body's many physiological changes, including temperature, airflow in the nose and mouth, respiration rate and volume, respiratory muscle function, chin muscle tone, eye movement, heart rate and rhythm, and oxygen content of the blood. In addition, your sleep may be videotaped under infrared light through a one-way mirror.

Is it actually possible to sleep under such conditions? Fortunately, yes. Polysomnography is painless and relatively free of discomfort. It involves no use of injections, anesthetics, or incisions. (In fact, as I have noted, some people actually sleep better in the lab than in their own homes, due to negative conditioning about sleeping in their familiar environment.) Although sleeping in such a strange place may seem disorienting or frightening, you may take comfort in the fact that trained professionals are keeping track of you at every point through intercoms and other means and will respond immediately if any problems occur.

If a night in the lab seems to have been problematical, a second night of polysomnography may be needed in order to overcome the effects of sleeping in such unusual surroundings.

When the polysomnograph recording is over, up to a half-mile of paper tracings will have been generated, listing the physical changes that have occurred throughout the entire night. The data provide a world of information, including

* sleep latency and duration
* type, severity, and pattern of sleep pathology (leg jerks, breathing disruptions)
* clues about other possible organic causes of insomnia (arrhythmias, etc.)
* patterns of sleeping and waking
* length of arousals and time needed to fall back asleep
* effects of sleeping position on the sleep pattern
* relative percentages of time spent in each sleep stage
* relationship of sleep disturbance to sleep stages

In addition, you will be asked for your subjective impressions about the quality and pattern of your sleep. These impressions will then be compared with the objective clinical findings. This is an extremely important step in assessing the nature of your complaint and how it affects your perception of sleep.

The complete body of information is delivered to your physician, who will then determine what course of action should be taken. One other important function of the sleep lab data is to provide a baseline for comparison in the future, which helps in measuring and assessing the effectiveness of therapeutic choices.

How much does such a procedure cost? Prices vary, depending on the region of the country, but the price tag for an initial examination plus a night in the lab is probably around $700. As I mentioned, a second night may also be needed, which could add another $400 to $500 to the cost. Rules for reimbursement from insurance companies for such services vary widely from state to state and even within insurers; I suggest that you contact your carrier before agreeing to undergo a lab evaluation.

One alternative to the sleep lab is the multiple sleep latency test, or MSLT. Conducted by a physician during the day, the MSLT involves recording five different nap periods of about twenty minutes in length, separated by an hour and forty minutes of wakefulness. With these repeated measurements the physician can assess the time it takes you to fall asleep and can detect the stages of sleep that occur soon after dropping off. MSLT is often used to distinguish patients with sleep apnea from those with narcolepsy; both fall asleep quickly when offered the opportunity to nap, but narcoleptics enter the REM stage almost immediately, while those with breathing disturbances seldom do. MSLT is considered more economical than a sleep lab evaluation; the cost averages about $400. Some insurance companies may be more willing to reimburse the costs of an MSLT than of a polysomnograph.

Of course, the ideal method would ultimately be to monitor your own sleep, unobtrusively, in your own bedroom environment. Advances in technology may make such an approach possible. Devices already exist to record blood pressure and heart rhythm on a twenty-four-hour basis. Recently a portable EEG was developed which uses a cassette recorder to store magnetic signals on four channels. The signals can then be played back on a video monitor or polygraph machine. While less complete than a lab-based EEG, the signals nonetheless can detect between 75 and 100 percent of any abnormal brain patterns needed to diagnose mental disturbance.

If you have been treated for insomnia for a significant period of time and feel the therapy is not working, discuss with your doctor the possibility of visiting a sleep lab. You may wish to contact the Association of Sleep Disorders Clinics (main office: 604 Second St. SW, Rochester, MN 55902) for further information.

11

Drug Therapy for Insomnia

The more we learn about sleep, the more we know about how to manage sleep disorders. In recent years, as data from sleep labs and other sources have become increasingly available, many physicians have begun to realize that in most cases pharmaceutical management of insomnia is at best a *temporary* solution. As a result of our growing knowledge, there has been a decided change in the way doctors deal with the problem. In 1964, the first year such data were collected, over 32 million prescriptions for sleeping pills were written. By 1971 the number peaked at over 42 million; by 1982, however, that figure had been cut exactly in half.

Throughout this book I have tried to make the point that insomnia is largely a symptom of an underlying medical or psychological problem. "Treating" insomnia by administering medicine may produce sleep for a few days or a few weeks, and the careful use of drugs can help especially if you are severely troubled by your insomnia or if inadequate sleep poses a threat to your health, safety, or well-being. However, unless your doctor uncovers the physical or mental disorder that is causing your sleeplessness, the problem will simply persist. In a sense sleeping pills are like throat lozenges, which soothe the irritation but do not cure the cough. No pill yet conceived cures insomnia. A more effective approach to chronic insomnia, as I explained in Chapter 10, is some combination of psychological and behavioral therapies, the goal of which is to encourage poor sleepers to quit dwelling on the symptoms and bring about changes in sleep habits.

There is one exception to the rule: in rare cases of true organic insomnia—sleeplessness without any identifiable medical or psychological cause—long-term therapy with sleep-inducing drugs may be required. Even then, treatment is most effective if the patient takes frequent drug "holidays," or respites, from the use of medication.

From the pharmaceutical fact file:

* Sleeping medications are the most widely used class of drugs in this country.
* Doctors write between 20 and 30 million prescriptions a year for sleeping pills and tranquilizers.
* Americans spend over $200 million a year for sleeping medications.
* Over 4 percent of the population—nearly 11 million people—use prescription sleep medicines.
* An even larger group uses over-the-counter preparations.
* About half of all patients in hospitals receive sleep medications at some point during their stay.
* Approximately 600 tons of sleeping medications are consumed each year.

Here's the kicker:

* In many cases these pills don't work, make the problem worse, or result in serious side effects. About a third of drug-related deaths reported to the Department of Health and Human Services involve sleeping pills.

THE EVOLUTION OF INSOMNIA DRUG THERAPY

For the first half of this century, barbiturates were the only pharmacological option available for insomnia. Veronal, the first barbiturate, was introduced in 1903. In the years following, about fifty drugs of this class reached the market (out of nearly twenty-five hundred barbiturate compounds developed in the lab). However, barbiturates were found to have two dangerous drawbacks: a high potential for addiction and a great risk of lethal overdose. Today only a dozen or so are still available; those used primarily for sleep are secobarbital (Seconal), amobarbital (combined with secobarbital in a product called Tuinal), and pentobarbital (Nembutal). Other uses for barbiturates are as antianxiety agents, anesthetics, and anticonvulsants.

In the late 1950s tricyclic antidepressants came on the market. In addition to their effect on serious depression, some of these drugs also possess sedative effects, although just how they work is not completely understood. Antidepressants offered an alternative to the potential dangers of barbiturates, but they too have undesirable side effects. While not considered the drug of first choice today, antidepressants may be used to alleviate insomnia—especially if the insomnia is associated with depression.

A major breakthrough in the drug treatment of insomnia was achieved with the arrival of benzodiazepines in the early 1960s. Compared to their prescription drug predecessors, benzodiazepines—primarily flurazepam, temazepam, and triazolam—have a greatly improved safety profile and are much more effective, particularly in disorders of initiating and maintaining sleep in individuals whose insomnia lacks an identifiable physical cause. Their improved ratio of therapeutic dose to lethal dose means a much lower risk of abuse or dangerous adverse effects. Some research does indicate, however, that there is a potential for addiction in patients taking the drugs over long periods of time. Benzodiazepines fall into several subcategories, usually depending on how quickly and for how long the drug works.

Of course, there are also several nonprescription sleeping aids available (brand names include Nytol, Sominex, and Sleep-Eze).

In all of these the active ingredient is the same: diphenhydramine, a form of antihistamine. As you may know, antihistamines are used to dry up secretions in the eyes, nose, and throat, thus relieving some symptoms of colds and allergies. The drowsiness caused by antihistamines is really only a side effect; makers of over-the-counter sleeping aids have thus taken a drug liability and marketed it as an asset. Antihistamines may prove especially useful in the treatment of insomnia complicated by a history of drug or alcohol abuse, since they do not have the potential for abuse that is associated with other drug therapies (such as benzodiazepines and barbiturates).

Other nonprescription sleep products contain a variety of ingredients, none of which is considered to be very effective. As a rule, then, I am not enthusiastic about the use of these products in insomnia. Besides being ineffective, especially in long-term use, they can cause nausea, vomiting, and other side effects; severe overdose can lead to coma and cardiorespiratory collapse. Antihistamines can also precipitate attacks of asthma in susceptible individuals.

Recently a consensus has emerged among physicians concerned with sleep disorders as to the appropriate stages of drug strategy for insomnia. Benzodiazepines are the drugs of first choice in the treatment of uncomplicated insomnia. Selection of the specific benzodiazepine depends on many factors, perhaps the most important being the duration of the drug's effects on the body. Using the drug for only a few days or weeks or taking the pills intermittently—say, on one night out of three—is prudent, because it poses the lowest risk of adverse effects while allowing the doctor to assess the overall effects of the drug and switch quickly to another if necessary. If the benzodiazepine appears not to be working, the option is to switch to another type of drug with sedative effects—for example, an antidepressant such as amitriptyline. Benzodiazepines are not used in patients who are already taking some other medication with sedative side effects, such as antidepressants or antihypertensives. Whatever the choice, long-term drug therapy in most cases should be avoided even if sleep has improved, so that other therapies can be tried.

Statistically, about 60 percent of the prescriptions for sleep medicines are for benzodiazepine hypnotic drugs (two thirds of which are for flurazepam); the rest are for antianxiety drugs, antidepressants, barbiturates, or the catch-all category known as nonbenzodiazepine, nonbarbiturate hypnotics. Roughly three out of four patients take medication for two weeks or less; one in ten, however, continues drug therapy for a year or more.

Hypnotics are prescribed for the elderly at a much higher rate than for other age groups, a rate far out of proportion to their actual numbers in the general population. For example, in 1975, although people over the age of sixty accounted for only 14 percent of the population, they received up to 45 percent of prescriptions for hypnotics. In nursing homes the number of residents given hypnotics ranges from 26 percent to 100 percent.

As we have seen, however, drugs are not always properly prescribed; due to the complex and confusing nature of insomnia, pharmacological management is often mishandled. According to government statistics, for example, about 30 percent of sleeping pill prescriptions are given to people whose problem is primarily psychological in origin; another 25 percent go to those with medical conditions that won't respond to sleeping pills, while still another 18 percent go to patients with ill-defined or vague symptoms that usually don't require drug treatment. Accepting these figures, then, we find that *as many as four out of five sleeping pill prescriptions are inappropriate or ineffective.*

Following is an overview of sleeping drugs and their effects. For a detailed compendium see the Appendix.

BENZODIAZEPINES

Flurazepam

As I mentioned, almost two out of three prescriptions for hypnotic benzodiazepines are written for flurazepam. Flurazepam was introduced in 1970 under the brand name Dalmane as the first and only drug in this class marketed in the United States as a hypnotic agent. Flurazepam reduces the time it takes to fall asleep; its hypnotic effect is felt within about fifteen to twenty minutes. The drug helps prevent nighttime arousals and reduces the time spent awake should an arousal occur. Like other benzodiazepines, flurazepam reduces deep sleep and increases sleep in Stage 2. The percentage of REM sleep is unchanged, but total sleep time increases.

It has a long half-life, ranging from forty to sixty hours. Because it is eliminated from the body so slowly, its effect can last well into the next day, a feature appropriate for patients who require daytime sedation but considered to be a side effect (known as drug hangover) in others, who may complain of decreased alertness or diminished coordination. Flurazepam seems to be effective for longer periods—up to four weeks—than most other benzodiazepines, which begin to lose their effectiveness with a few days or weeks. However, the drug accumulates in the body to the point where there is as much of the compound circulating in the bloodstream during the day as there is at night; its hypnotic effect persists for a day or more following cessation of therapy. Because the elderly eliminate drugs from their system at a much slower rate, they should be given flurazepam only with great caution; I usually prescribe half the usual dose for a patient over sixty-five. If the drug is not used properly in older patients, it can create side effects that appear to be (but are not) symptoms of organic psychosis, such as confusion and agitation.

Temazepam

Sold as Restoril, temazepam is especially appropriate for people whose insomnia takes the form of middle-of-the-night awakenings, because its half-life of about ten hours means the drug stays effective throughout the period of sleep. On a temporary basis some people may be able to take a temazepam pill as needed after a nighttime awakening to help facilitate a return to sleep, with only a relatively small risk that the sedative effects will persist into the morning. However, the drug is absorbed slowly in the gastrointestinal tract; some people thus find it ineffective in helping them fall asleep unless taken an hour or two before bedtime. Temazepam does prevent nighttime awakenings, and it improves the duration and subjective quality of sleep. Some physicians may also use temazepam to treat cases of nocturnal myoclonus or restless legs, although this is not an approved indication for the drug.

Triazolam

Marketed under the brand name Halcion, triazolam possesses the shortest half-life (four to six hours) of the major hypnotic benzodiazepines; thus the effects of the drug are usually completely gone by morning. It is especially useful in cases of transient insomnia, or for occasional use in chronic insomnia when sedative or antianxiety effects are not appropriate. With triazolam the onset of sleep occurs more quickly; REM sleep is delayed, but the total percentage of REM sleep is not affected. Sleep time is longer, but there is less deep sleep; there are also fewer awakenings. Triazolam has other uses as well; it can help to manage the disruptive behaviors in sleep-disturbed patients with Alzheimer's. Furthermore, as I mentioned earlier, it may help overcome the symptoms of jet lag by causing rapid adjustments of the biological clock. Triazolam is more rapidly absorbed than temazepam, but it poses the risk of a number of side effects, including early-morning insomnia, memory impairment, psychotic symptoms, sleepwalking activity, and rebound insomnia if withdrawal from the drug is not handled properly.

Other Benzodiazepines

The drugs just discussed are indicated primarily for the treatment of insomnia. Other benzodiazepines possess other qualities, such as relief of the anxiety and depression that may be associated with insomnia. Some induce amnesia, which can actually be a beneficial property in controlled circumstances—for example, when it is desirable for a patient to forget the unpleasant feelings associated with cancer chemotherapy. Perhaps the most well known benzodiazepine is diazepam, sold under the brand name Valium and widely used in the treatment of anxiety. Some physicians treating patients with Valium may decide to use the drug for insomnia, perhaps by altering the time of administration. If such an approach fails, other drugs such as flurazepam or temazepam may prove effective. In some cases, lorazepam (Ativan) or quazepam (Dormalin) may help a patient's sleeplessness.

ANTIDEPRESSANTS

As their name suggests, antidepressants are used primarily in the treatment of depression. For this reason, and because of the possibility of side effects, they are not generally used for patients with chronic insomnia. However, in depressed patients antidepressants may provide effective treatment of both the insomnia and the depression, making the patients feel more hopeful and less helpless, which in turn can make them more responsive to other forms of therapy.

Tricyclic antidepressants are the most widely used drugs for treatment of depression. The tricyclics possess varying degrees of sedative effect; amitriptyline (Elavil) and doxepin (Sinequan) are the most sedating, whereas protriptyline and desipramine may actually cause the patient to feel more energetic. Imipramine is sometimes used to manage parasomnias (such as sleepwalking and bed-wetting). These drugs, and others called monoamine oxidase inhibitors (MAOIs) used in the treatment of depression, appear to work at least in part by increasing the amount of certain chemical messengers in the brain, including those responsible for sleep. In addition, or perhaps as a consequence, they tend to suppress REM sleep; such suppression may in itself produce some therapeutic benefits. Often the sedative effect of an antidepressant will appear in a very short time—a day or two—whereas the impact on depression may not be noticed for weeks.

Of course, these powerful drugs may produce side effects, ranging from dry mouth, sweating, and constipation to more severe problems such as cardiotoxicity and arrhythmias. In situations where it becomes important to reduce anxiety and manage depression at the same time, benzodiazepines can be used along with tricyclics without risking harmful interactions. However, tricyclics can interfere with the actions of antihypertensive medications. One further complication of using sedating antidepressants is that their effects often occur during the daytime, thus causing the patient to struggle with sleepiness while trying to function on the job or in other settings. Changing the regimen so that more drug is taken at night than in the morning can help.

New antidepressants continue to come onto the market. One

goal of new drugs is to improve efficacy while reducing side effects; consequently, these "second generation" antidepressants may have fewer sedative effects and thus may not generally be considered as valid therapeutic options in the treatment of insomnia.

As I mentioned earlier, the use of the EEG to detect onset of REM sleep in depressed patients is proving to be an effective way to measure the results of therapy with tricyclic medications. For example, amitriptyline and other tricyclics such as desipramine are known to produce rapid suppression of REM sleep as measured by delays in onset of REM, reduction of the intensity of REM activity, and decrease in the overall percentage of time spent in REM sleep. Thus if REM is found to occur soon after onset of sleep, the patient's response to the drug is thought to be inadequate. Future studies will help define, and refine, the use of this valuable diagnostic tool.

BARBITURATES

The use of barbiturates for sleep has all but disappeared in recent years. In 1971 these drugs accounted for 47 percent of the prescriptions for hypnotic medications; six years later the figure had dropped to 17 percent, and by 1982 it was 9 percent. That the figure is even this high has more to do with entrenched prescribing habits among some physicians than with appropriate choice of therapy. One reason for the decline is the high risk of tolerance, dependence, and addiction involved with the use of barbiturates. Besides, such drugs as Seconal and Nembutal lose their effectiveness quickly, compelling users to step up the dosage.

Barbiturates can be deadly drugs; a dosage only fifteen times higher than that needed for sleep can be fatal. In the past barbiturates were the drugs most frequently used in suicide attempts. The presence of alcohol greatly increases the danger; even relatively small doses of barbiturates and alcohol can be fatal. Furthermore, the liver deterioration that accompanies alcoholism means that heavy drinkers are at special risk if they also use barbiturates because these toxic drugs must be broken down in the liver. These drugs may actually worsen sleep by suppressing the deep NREM and REM stages. And during withdrawal from medication, sleep can be even worse than before use of the drug and is marked by REM rebound, hallucinations, anxiety, or, in severe cases, seizures.

OTHER DRUGS USED IN INSOMNIA

Chloral Hydrate

Sold as Noctec, chloral hydrate is one of the ingredients, along with alcohol, of the knockout drink known as a Mickey Finn. This drug is used for patients unable to take other types of prescription sleep medicines, such as the very young, the very old, and the very ill. Since the creation of benzodiazepines chloral hydrate is used less frequently, although physicians concerned about flurazepam's long half-life may opt to prescribe chloral hydrate instead. Noctec is relatively inexpensive and the risk of overdosage or side effects, such as gastric irritation, is low.

Glutethimide; Methyprylon

Originally, these drugs were offered as alternative sedatives to barbiturates, but they were found to have actions similar to the drugs they were meant to replace—and similar drawbacks as well, including the potential for addiction. Many physicians feel the hazards so far outweigh any possible benefit that they will not prescribe these drugs under any circumstances.

Ethchlorvynol

Known by the brand name Placidyl, ethchlorvynol is unrelated to other hypnotic drugs. Its advantages are primarily that it is absorbed quickly and that it has a half-life of only six hours, resulting in a lower risk of daytime sedation. The drug improves the onset of sleep, but its effects wear off during the middle of the night, and it will be effective only for a few days at a time. Side effects include confusion and emotional distress on the following day, as well as lack of coordination, confusion, slurred speech, and muscle weakness; there is also a strong potential for inducing drug-withdrawal insomnia.

Methysergide Maleate

Generally indicated for the treatment of vascular headache, this drug, sold under the brand name Sansert, has some use in the treatment of excessive daytime sleepiness of undetermined cause. Symptoms of this disorder include prolonged sleep and sleep drunkenness, but without the other symptoms of narcolepsy, such as cataplexy.

Tryptophan

Tryptophan is not a drug and is thus not subject to regulation or testing by the FDA. It is an essential amino acid that is derived from the protein found in foods such as grains, legumes, and seeds. Tryptophan is also sold as a dietary supplement in health food stores and drugstores. Many believe tryptophan may play a role in facilitating the onset of sleep through its effects on the production of serotonin (see page 175 for more information).

CONCERNS OF DRUG THERAPY

While the list of medications available for the management of sleep disorders seems long, I hope I have made the point that none of these remedies is without potential side effects or problems that may affect their use. A summary of some of the common problems associated with drug therapy reads like a "Ten Most Unwanted" list in medical management.

* Tolerance, reliance, dependence, addiction
* Worsening of sleep patterns (rebound or withdrawal insomnia)
* Negative effect on sleep cycle (REM and NREM effects)
* Amnesia
* Impaired daytime functioning (drowsiness, inability to concentrate)

* Toxic effects on the heart and other organ systems (kidney, liver, respiration)
* Hallucinations, confusion, other psychosis
* Complications of pregnancy
* Risk of interactions with other drugs
* Death

As one sleep researcher put it, many of these pills don't really improve the ability to sleep; they merely inhibit the ability to stay awake. What's more, some physicians feel that there is no evidence to suggest that people are better off during the daytime just because they were able to sleep after taking medication. Obviously, any lasting effects on personality or outlook on life are more likely to arise as a result of some kind of psychotherapy.

The bottom line: if you suffer from insomnia, don't run to your doctor demanding a prescription for a sleeping pill. Remember that the use of drugs, if indicated at all, is a temporary solution and one fraught with hazards and complications. By availing yourself of the various nonpharmacological therapeutic options, you give yourself the greatest chance of enjoying a good night's sleep—not just tonight but for many nights to come.

12

The Other Side of Sleep: Dreams and Nightmares

THE ROLE OF DREAMING

If I were to ask you to describe the dream you had just before waking up this morning, you would probably respond in one of two ways: either you would say you don't remember the dream, or you would grope for words adequate to express the bizarre events and oblique emotional feelings the dream portrayed. Then as you continue to relate the dream, you would probably sense that even as you speak, what little clarity it might have possessed is slipping away from your grasp, dissolving like a chalk drawing on a rain-soaked sidewalk.

Why do we dream? Why for nearly two hours a night do we become citizens of a kingdom where, as in Alice's Wonderland, the familiar is strange and logic seems to have been banished by some insane royal decree? Does dreaming serve some deeply rooted biological need by allowing us tantalizing but mystifying glimpses of the inner workings of our minds? Or is it, as some propose, merely the random firings of neurons in the brain as it processes—and disposes of—the day's emotional debris? Such questions have been asked since consciousness first dawned inside the human skull.

A Dream History

For centuries dreams were thought to be messages, not always benevolent, whispered by the gods who wished to warn, instruct, or manipulate humans for their own mysterious purposes. For example, the ancient Egyptians believed that if a woman dreamed of kissing her husband, she was headed for trouble; if she dreamed of intercourse with a goat, she was about to die. In many ancient societies the diviners who could interpret dreams held power, perhaps second only to kings and queens themselves, because they represented the link between the gods and the people below. During biblical times, for instance, Joseph became an Egyptian hero because he interpreted Pharaoh's dreams as foretelling seven years of starvation; by laying in stores of food, the people were saved.

The ancient Greeks took dreams very seriously, regarding them as real events occurring in an alternate world. Besides their power to predict the future, dreams were thought to hold the key to illness. Hippocrates, for example, interpreted them as diagnostic clues to his patients' problems: a dream of a river meant he should check the blood for signs of disease; a tree was a signal to examine the reproductive system. Aesculapius, the god of healing, was believed to appear to afflicted people in their dreams, effecting his cures as they slept. Plato referred to the "lawless wild-beast nature" of the human species which peers out while we sleep. Aristotle denied the divine origin of dreams; dismissing them as the remnants of sensory impressions, he thought of them merely as accidents, like the eddies and ripples seen in the flowing water of a river.

The first systematic treatise on dream interpretation, written by a Greek-speaking resident of Asia Minor named Artemidorus, appeared in the second century A.D. Artemidorus put his stock in dreams as portents of the future. Other cultures held—and still hold, for that matter—that dreams represent visits from the dead or are brief sojourns into other worlds undertaken by our disembodied souls.

In the nineteenth century, philosophers held widely divergent views on the role of dreaming. Some decried dreams as pointless and irritating, describing them as psychological activity that is "transported from the brain of a reasonable man into that of a fool"; others looked on them as nothing more than a degradation of the intellectual and rational capacity of the mind. Immanuel Kant ascribed an important biological role to dreams, believing them responsible for stimulating and regulating the function of "vital organs" such as the digestive system. (Conversely, Dickens's Scrooge attributes the appearance of Marley's ghost to a "fragment of an underdone potato" or an "undigested bit of beef"—"There's more of gravy than of grave about you whatever you are," he chuckles.) Nietzsche believed passionately that dreams were an integral part of our psychological makeup, exclaiming that "nothing contains more of your own work than your dreams! Nothing belongs to you so much!"

Freud and Dreams

In modern times the renewed argument over the function of dreams was triggered primarily by the pioneering work of Sigmund Freud, whose *The Interpretation of Dreams* was published in 1900. Freud considered dreams to be a special language of the mind, one in which repressed sexual desires arising from our childhood relationships with our parents are expressed, and therefore fulfilled, in symbolic fashion. Dreams thus serve as a form of safety valve through which we may discharge mental and emotional conflict; yet dreams protect our psyches (and our sleep) by disguising the wish in such a way as to prevent us from waking with feelings of shame, guilt, or alarm.

Dreams, said Freud, operate on two levels of meaning: the "manifest" level, made up of the specific images and details as reported by the dreamer, and the "latent" level, containing all the hidden associations and meanings that can be revealed and interpreted only through the process of careful, thorough psychoanalysis. The events depicted in dreams are drawn from actual events that occurred while the dreamer was awake; these events are somehow selected for inclusion by the dreaming mind because they can be connected or associated in some way with events or complexes buried deep within the psyche. Before appearing in the dream, however, the events undergo a process called dream work, involving some kind of transformation or censorship so that their true, and presumably horrifying, nature is disguised from our conscious perception. As his work progressed, Freud became convinced that certain symbols or themes that appeared in a dream held special meaning for the individual dreamer, and that an understanding of the associations each person makes with the symbols was required in order to grasp the significance of the dream. Thus, in the process of analysis, the dreamer is asked to associate freely on the various elements of the dream and their possible connection to other events in the past. Wrote Freud, "The interpretation of dreams is in fact the royal road to a knowledge of the unconscious."

Interestingly, although much of Freud's work was devoted to the study of the important revelations that he perceived in his patients' dreams, he believed that a sleep without dreams is the best—indeed, the only—desirable kind of sleep. Subsequent developments in the field of psychiatry departed from this view. For example, Carl Jung, a student and onetime disciple of Freud, held that dreams revealed not just the root of the neurosis but its prognosis and treatment as well. For Jung, dreams contained the whole range of human experience since the race began—everything from fantasy, memory, and foresight to telepathic insights and glimpses of transcendental truths.

The Dream Debate

Today, with the increased attention paid to sleep by the medical community, the debate over the function of dreams continues apace. As in any good debate, there are opposing schools of thought, each armed with volumes of data to prove its points. One camp, comprised mainly of psychiatrists and psychologists, stands committed to the belief, inherited from Freud, that dreams serve a largely psychological function by revealing our hidden natures. Another camp, made up largely of investigators from such hard-science disciplines as biology and neurology, believes dreams are merely electrical and chemical phenomena, no more meaningful than the random swirling patterns of light and color you see when you press firmly on your closed eyelids. Somewhere in the middle is another faction, which adopts the view that a certain neurological randomness may indeed trigger the process of dreaming, but that the images and sensations evoked may be tied together in such a way as to hold some psychological meaning for the dreamer.

One reason for the existence of such divergent views stems from the fact that some of Freud's work has been largely discredited since its initial publication. For example, Freud declared that the dreams of neurotic people do not differ in any significant way from those of normal people. Subsequent research has determined that the dreams of the mentally disturbed do reflect the underlying condition: anxious people dream about their anxieties; phobic people dream about their phobias. The dreams of people suffering from depression focus on themes of violence or the failure to repair damage of some kind, while the dreams of schizophrenics are filled with images of catastrophe and devastation in remote places. The notion that REM sleep deprivation provides therapeutic benefits in the treatment of depression tends to undermine Freud's theory that dreaming serves as an essential psychological safety valve.

Discoveries in brain physiology—new understanding of the structure and functioning of the brain, information not available to Freud—also make it difficult for some scientists to accept his concepts of dreaming. One school of thought holds, for example, that the very processes at work in the sleeping brain are themselves directly responsible for dream activity. In this model the activity of rapid eye movement is believed to stimulate the neural pathways that connect the eyes to the brain. Such stimulation directly affects the motor regions of the brain, in turn generating dream images of movement; it can also affect the forebrain, thus triggering memories or causing feelings of emotion to enter the dream picture. This theory, however, fails to account for the fact that dreaming occurs, to one extent or another, in all stages of sleep—a fact I'll expand on shortly.

During REM sleep the brain experiences a firestorm of electrical activity, which some scientists refer to as the "dream state generator." Originating in the pons ("bridge"), a structure that spans the gap between the midbrain and the medulla, this electrical activity spreads over the cerebral cortex, the structure responsible for thought and motor activity. The bizarre and random nature of dreams reflects the randomness of the electrical discharge. Obviously, the theories of Freud can be dispensed with in a scientific model that portrays dreams merely as arbitrary accumulations of images, like a scrambled television signal. Some investigators, however, carry the "dream generator" concept a step further. According to this school of thought, the creation of visual and auditory hallucinations may indeed be a random process. The actual dream, however, is the process by which the cortex tries to weave unconnected images, sounds, and feelings into some kind of meaningful fabric. Our unconscious wishes, then, may serve as the loom on which this fabric is woven. Contrary to Freud's view, these wishes do not actually cause the dream, but they exploit the existence of confused signals by imposing their own order upon them.

Other dream research focuses on the role of dreaming in organizing and storing memories. In this model, dreams are a way of reexperiencing the events of the day so that they can be consolidated, organized into patterns, and placed in storage. People who espouse this view use an analogy drawn from the world of computers: dreams are a form of software that takes a "short-term" memory, processes it, and files it in "long-term" memory. To accommodate the Freudian view, some experts feel that dreams serve to "match" new events with old items already stored in memory—from our childhoods, say—so as to form meaningful patterns and incorporate new experiences into a broader "data base."

The noted researcher Francis Crick and his colleague Graeme Mitchison take a radically different view: they believe dreams help us to forget. The random electrical activity in the cortex during REM sleep serves to erase useless information, much as a degausser will erase an entire audiotape with the flick of a button. This form of electrical housecleaning, they hypothesize, enables us to get by with smaller and more efficient brains than we would otherwise need if we retained every sight, sound, and thought we had ever encountered. Without such a system our brains would resemble crowded library shelves. It would be harder to locate the precise information we are searching for, and similar thoughts might become confused during the retrieval process. In this concept the jumbled pictures that appear to us in dreams are merely the meaningless accidents of the unlearning process. The notion that we dream to forget may also help explain why it is so difficult to remember our dreams.

There are other schools of thought as well. According to some experts, dreams facilitate learning by forging new branches of association between previously unrelated thoughts or images. Others believe that dreams help us adapt to and deal with threatening experiences we have sidestepped or sublimated during the day, perhaps by enabling us to discharge instinctual drives, such as fear and aggression, which are inappropriate during our more "civilized" waking hours. Taking their cue from Hippocrates, a group of Soviet scientists claims to have found evidence that dreams, when properly interpreted, can serve as predictors of disease when conventional medical tests have failed.

Which of these views, if any, is right? Only time and further research will tell. Until all the facts are in (an event that may never occur), it seems to me the wisest position to hold is one that incorporates elements from several theories and synthesizes them into the broadest possible interpretation. Perhaps, then, dreams serve many functions. They reduce psychic tensions by discharging them in a relatively harmless fashion during a time when our brains are otherwise unoccupied by conscious thought. In the process they dispose of unnecessary information or potentially harmful feelings and fears, thus wiping the slate so that the brain can then rearrange short-term memories and incorporate them as part of long-term storage. By clearing the shelves in our brain's library of outdated information, dreams may prepare us for the new set of sensory and intellectual encounters that await us when next we wake.

THE MEANING OF DREAMS

As is the case with many aspects of sleep research, there is no real answer to the question of why we dream. But what about the content of dreams? Is a dream a subconscious "letter to oneself," filled with cryptic instructions on how to cope with life? Or is it merely a garbled instant replay of the day's events, with no structure or meaning? Any answer given by medical scientists will naturally reflect their concept of the origin of dreams. Those who see dreams as a purely physical, biological process will completely discount the significance of content and thus may overlook clues to the functioning of consciousness. On the other hand, those who see them as indispensable keys to personality are perhaps prone to imbue them with far more meaning than they actually contain.

That many dreams are connected to the past day's events is obvious. You probably recall your own dreams in which you rehashed a recent confrontation or replayed characters or scenes from the movie you watched before going to bed. These incidents are usually transformed; they might take place in an unfamiliar house, for example, or a person in the dream might have the face of a close friend but play an altogether different relational role— as a parent or sibling, perhaps. It is these very transformations or associations that intrigue psychiatrists and others, who wonder why the brain bothers to make the changes instead of just replaying the scene uncut, unrevised, and uncensored.

Investigators who have studied thousands of dream reports find that very few dreams actually contain bizarre and fantastic elements, although such dreams are the ones more likely to be remembered. Most dreams are, in fact, quite ordinary. As a rule, at least one familiar person will appear in virtually every dream. In one out of three dreams, the "star" of the show (most often ourselves, but frequently the familiar person) will be moving in some way—walking, perhaps, or traveling in some vehicle or other. Routine activities, such as housework or office tasks, are seldom depicted. In some cases movement is difficult or impossible, as though the dreamer was trying to jog through molasses. Usually, however, physical effort is easily achieved. Researchers have also studied the effect of immediate sensory stimulation on dreams. For example, in one experiment, sleeping subjects were sprinkled with water and then awakened thirty seconds later. Some (but not all) of the subjects reported dreams that involved water in some way.

Some people have recurring dreams, which need not necessarily be nightmares; others have what could be called progressive dreams. One of my patients, a woman in her forties, reported a sequence of dreams that have unfolded over a period of decades (and which continue to unfold). In the first dream, which occurred around the age of ten, she attempted to fly by flapping her arms; although the work was exhausting, she eventually managed to skim over the ground (not without suffering a few bumps and bruises along the way). In subsequent dreams, however, the flying became more and more effortless. During her most recent dream, she said, she was teaching and giving public demonstrations of her flying, swooping above the heads of awed spectators in arenas and convention halls.

Somewhat surprisingly, two out of three dreams of healthy people are reported to have negative or unpleasant content, including feelings of anger, sadness, defeat, failure, or fear. While these might be considered "bad" dreams, they are entirely different in origin and impact from nightmares, as we will see shortly. In bad dreams, acts of physical or verbal hostility directed against the dreamer predominate, outnumbering friendly acts by a ratio of two to one. However, the feelings one has on waking after one of these dreams do not usually correspond to the intensity of the dream situation. Naturally, some bad dreams are directly related to situational stress, personal loss, or grief. That such stress can disrupt sleep, and consequently dreams, is one concept on which sleep researchers agree. The disruption—as measured by REM onset and duration—can be short-term, or it can persist for decades.

To a limited extent, your gender can also affect the content of your dreams. Generalizations are tricky, but as a rule men will dream more often about other men than about women; women will dream about both sexes in roughly equal measure. Predictably, men's dreams involve physical activity and aggression; women tend to emphasize emotional themes, and their dreams contain more conversations. The events in women's dreams (and, according to some research, in the dreams of male homosexuals) are likelier to occur indoors than outside. In studies of children, boys more often mention dreams involving use of tools and other objects, while the dreams of girls are more likely to be populated with people than things.

Sexual dreams occur only about 1 percent of the time. As stated earlier, nocturnal penile tumescence and clitoral stimulation are functions of circadian and other rhythms and are not necessarily connected to the content of dreams. Notwithstanding, many dreams do of course contain sexual elements. One sensible theory is that the brain, reacting to signals of arousal, may then incorporate those responses into the dream pattern. If this is the case, then an erotic dream may be thought of as an effect, not a cause, of sexual stimulation during sleep. (I remember one patient who told me that, as a boy, he would often study the centerfold from a *Playboy* magazine, then close his eyes, turn out the light, and climb into bed. His theory—and his hope—was that the last image he saw before turning in would appear in his dreams. The experiment, he reported, was not successful.)

At this point we are left with yet another unanswered question: do dreams have meaning? For many people, and for many medical professionals, they do. I would be foolish to ignore the dreams reported to me by my patients; if nothing else, such reports serve to throw light on themes, topics, or areas of concern to the individual. If a patient is troubled by recurring dreams of death or physical violence, for example, I may indeed discover, through careful questioning, that he or she has suffered some personal loss or trauma that is affecting the ability to sleep. The very fact that people remember one particular dream and not another may indicate areas of sensitivity that weigh heavily on their minds. Conversely, I am not inclined to believe that every single dream experienced by every person on every night is crammed with significance. Many dreams may indeed be nothing more than neurological twitchings that occur when other brain functions have been curtailed for the night. One interesting area of research might be to see if random neuron firings similar to those of the dreaming state occur just as frequently during the day; such firings may be masked or may pass unnoticed because we are preoccupied with the conscious thoughts, emotions, and sensory experiences that fill our brains during the waking hours.

The Dream Diary

If you are curious about the meaning of your dreams, try keeping a dream diary (see accompanying box). Whenever you awaken during the night, immediately write down everything you can remember about your most recent dream—characters, events, settings, colors, sounds, and any emotional connotations you find. Eventually you may begin to discern a pattern which holds some particular significance for you. There are a number of dream dictionaries and other dream workbooks available that are intended to help you interpret your findings. I suggest, however, that you take such books with a large helping of salt. If

THE DREAM DIARY

Keeping a diary of your dreams provides a record of your nighttime adventures and can help you discover whether they hold some hidden meaning or significance. Such a journal may also prove useful if you participate in some form of psychiatric therapy. While you should write down your dream in as much detail as possible immediately after it happens, don't let the process of doing so interfere with your ability to get a good night's sleep. Write down the key elements of the plot, setting, and characters involved, as well as the emotions you experience. On rising in the morning, you might wish to expand on these in greater detail.

Among the questions you might want to address are:

* What is the predominant feeling you experience immediately after waking from the dream?
* Who appeared in the dream: Yourself? Friends? Family? Strangers? Animals? Monsters?
* What happened in the dream?
* Where did the events of the dream occur? Was the setting strange, familiar, indoors, outdoors?
* When did the dream occur (time of night as well as the time that appeared in the dream: day, night, past, present, future)?
* Can you explain why this particular dream might have occurred to you?
* Can you connect the events in the dream to events within (a) the past few hours; (b) the last twenty-four hours; (c) the past week or month; (d) the distant past?
* Do you recognize any images, symbols, events, or themes as having occurred in previous dreams?
* Do you remember any specific sounds or colors?

dreams have any meaning at all, such meaning is a very personal affair; you are the only person who can state whether a particular image is significant, based on your own experiences, feelings, and associations. As Nietzsche stated and as Freud himself believed, "nothing belongs to you so much" as your dreams.

SLEEP STAGES AND DREAM STAGES

Setting aside such controversial topics as the why and what of dreaming, we turn now to a more concrete field of exploration: the actual process involved with the mechanics—the how—of dreaming.

As you have no doubt noticed, the first step in the process of falling asleep—also called Stage 0—involves a usually pleasant mixture of diminishing consciousness and rising unconsciousness. During this time our awareness of the environment drops rapidly, although we remain somewhat sensitive to outside stimuli, such as sound. Soon we begin to lose control over our flow of thoughts. To demonstrate this, try an experiment: some night, as you begin to feel yourself drifting off to sleep, try to keep talking. Recite a poem, recount a fairy tale, or conduct a conversation. Listen carefully to yourself; you'll be surprised at the utterly unpredictable turns your speech takes. You may be reciting the Gettysburg Address, for example, and suddenly find yourself babbling about the ingredients of a favorite recipe. If someone stirs you during this later part of Stage 0, you may have trouble remembering where you are or what time it is.

In the next portion of Stage 0 you may experience dreamlike images, even before you have actually fallen asleep. During this phase you are no longer able to distinguish these images, technically known as hypnagogic hallucinations, from reality. In fact, sleep experts who study transcripts of dream reports from this phase are unable to distinguish them from reports taken after arousal from REM sleep. Dreams during Stage 0 tend to focus on experiences from the previous few hours. As you drift, you also experience feelings of weightlessness, loss of balance, or floating. You may experience sudden shudders or whole-body jerks; some researchers believe these are related to the release of tensions stored deep within the body.

Sleep actually begins at Stage 1, when EEG tracings reveal a distinctive pattern of brain waves. Dream activity can occur at this stage, and at all other stages of sleep for that matter. Studies have found that between 30 and 75 percent of the time, people aroused from the NREM phases of the sleep cycle report having dreams, especially during the early part of the night. Although visual displays can certainly occur, such dreams seem more logical and are usually described as vague or fragmentary "thoughts." However, NREM dreams occurring in the later part of the night are reported as being more "dreamlike." The nature of NREM dreams depends to some extent on the quality of your sleep; light sleepers, for example, report more NREM dreams than heavy sleepers. Evidence also suggests that in certain people, "dream spillover" into NREM stages may be related to some form of mental illness.

The ability to recall dreams is also related to sleep stages. Arousal to consciousness is more difficult during the NREM part of the cycle, and thus it is harder to recount a dream if you are awakened during slow-wave sleep. As we have seen, most people naturally awaken to a significant degree three or four times a night, following the completion of a REM period, and are therefore more likely to report dreams that occur during this phase.

REM and Dreams

Up to 85 percent of the total time spent in REM—nearly two hours out of a typical night's sleep for an adult—is spent dreaming. Children spend even more time in REM and thus more time in a dream state.

On entering the REM phase, the body undergoes a number of physiological changes. Erections occur, metabolism jumps, blood flow to the brain increases as much as 40 percent. Our kidneys manufacture less urine, but it is more concentrated. In many areas of the brain spontaneous electrical activity occurs at a higher rate than while we are awake. Normally such activity would trigger corresponding responses in our muscles; fortunately, as we have seen, a mechanism exists whereby such impulses are usually suppressed. Such paralysis, or atonia, is believed to arise from nerve cells in an area of the brain called the pons. (Freud, in fact, believed we are able to experience intense dreams, filled with forbidden feelings, only because of this benign nocturnal paralysis. However, as we will see, it is not present during NREM sleep; some people even lack the trait during REM sleep and are thus prone to act out their dreams—sometimes with violent consequences.) Research indicates that, in addition to motor activity, the nerve cells responsible for motivation and memory are also shut down during REM dreaming, which may account in part for the fact that dreams are involuntary and are so easily forgotten.

Although eye movement is the dominant feature of REM sleep, it is a matter of controversy whether the movements are actually associated with the content of dreams. Some researchers have found, for example, that people dreaming of such events as a Ping-Pong match shift their gaze from left to right, and evidence suggests that intense eye movements seem to correspond with shifts in focus in the dream as narrated by the dreamer after arousal. Other investigators, however, believe that no such connection exists between the content of a dream and the physical signs of dreaming. As evidence they cite the fact that people who have been blind since birth also exhibit rapid eye movement.

REM dreams usually contain more visual images than auditory ones; some researchers think this is because dreaming occurs primarily in the right brain, responsible for visual function, whereas the left brain, responsible for auditory function, is less involved. I should point out, though, that other experts feel dreaming is not centralized in a particular hemisphere, but involves the entire brain. People who were once able to see but have become blind retain the ability to "see" visual images in dreams for ten years or more after the loss of sight; this ability, however, ultimately fades. And yes, we do usually dream in color, although the presence or absence of color is not thought to hold any particular significance.

How Long Do Dreams Last?

Many people wonder how long a dream lasts. In the past it was thought that dreams occurred in a flash. Freud relates an anecdote that seems to support such a notion. A man reported having dreamed that, during the French Revolution, he was hauled before the authorities and condemned to death: decapitation by guillotine. He was summarily thrust into the fiendish device and watched in horror as the blade fell. He awakened to find that his bed had collapsed and the headboard was pressing against his neck. Dream experts note that the accident must have occurred in an instant, so the accompanying dream, apparently a subconscious—and quite imaginative—effort to alert the dreamer to the emergency, must likewise have taken place in a flash. Similarly, in Ambrose Bierce's fascinating tale "Occurrence at Owl Creek Bridge," a man about to be hanged fantasizes that he escapes the noose, flees his pursuers, and is reunited with his lover—all in the split second it takes him to fall through the trapdoor and feel the noose tighten about his neck.

Notwithstanding these stories, current research suggests that the length of dreams usually corresponds to the length of the REM phase—in other words, a twenty-minute REM period will produce a dream nearly twenty minutes long. This discovery was made by waking people at various points in the REM cycle and comparing their dream reports with the length of REM sleep. Interestingly, when sleepers are awakened after a very long REM period—up to fifty minutes or an hour, say—they report having the feeling that they dreamed for a long time but can remember only the last fifteen minutes or so of the dream. It thus appears that the process of forgetting our dreams begins even as the dream is taking place.

Children and Dreams

Earlier I mentioned the differences in content between the dreams of men and women. Your age also affects the way you dream, especially during childhood. Between the ages of two and three, for example, children do not report dreams as a rule. At four and five they may report dreams about 15 percent of the time; these dreams are somewhat like a scrapbook of photographs—still images with no story line, which appear briefly, usually feature animals rather than humans, and have little emotional content. From age five to seven the incidence of dreaming doubles to about 30 percent; dreams at this stage depict events in a series and feature physical and social activity with family and friends in familiar settings. Girls of this age are more likely to describe dreams involving friendly encounters, pleasant feelings, and happy endings; boys, on the other hand, have more unhappy dreams involving conflict. Not until ages eight and nine do dreams become animated, or more like a movie, with character, plot, and action, usually focusing on active participation by the dreamers. Gender differences in dream content are not discernible at this stage. About 43 percent of children of eight and nine report having dreams, compared to 80 percent of older children and adults. Dream recall declines with age, until by age 70 reports of dreams drop to about 43 percent.

NIGHTMARES

As we have seen, dreaming is a natural, universal, and in many ways perhaps even beneficial process. There are times, however, when our dreams are not so benign, when the images and feelings they generate disturb our sleep and cause emotional disruption that persists far into our waking hours. I refer, of course, to nightmares.

Etymologically, a "mare" in this context refers not to a horse but to a goblin or incubus, an evil spirit believed to have sexual intercourse with a sleeping woman. On a more clinical level, a nightmare is defined as a dream that occurs during a REM sleep period, usually lasts about twenty minutes, and provokes such intense anxiety that it causes the sleeper to awaken in a state of emotional distress. Nightmares, like other REM period dreams, are likely to be recalled by the dreamer, most often in very vivid detail. I need hardly describe the content of these dreams: scenes of falling, persecution, embarrassment, fear, violence, danger, death. Often the same theme recurs in the dreams of a particular individual. Approximately 5 percent of the adult population currently experiences difficulty with nightmares; another 5 percent have had problems with them in the past. The onset of nightmares usually occurs early in life; roughly 50 percent of my patients who report disturbing dreams have experienced them with some consistency since before the age of ten. Statistically an adult is likely to have at least one nightmare a year; only one person in five hundred has them as often as once a week. Recent research has confirmed the notion that those who suffer from frequent nightmares are likely to be the so-called creative types—painters, musicians, and writers. Women are apparently more susceptible than men to nightmares.

Because nightmares are so widespread, they are considered by some experts a normal, possibly even a healthy, part of growth and development. The ability to feel fear, for example, is thought to be an inborn and largely positive trait. Such instincts warn us of danger and prompt us to act to remove ourselves from it.

Nightmare Triggers

Nightmares are often triggered by stress and trauma. For example, studies focusing on combat veterans, victims of accidents or disasters, and Holocaust survivors find a high incidence of disturbed dreams, which are directly linked to the subjects' past experiences. Such dreams can persist for decades after the actual event; the severity of their impact is directly related to the time that has passed since the trauma occurred. In one such study victims of a disaster at sea were found to relive the crisis on an almost nightly basis. Their REM periods were fragmented and interrupted; during their dreams of the disaster, they would cry out in fear and move about so violently that they sometimes fell out of bed. A man who had survived the Holocaust at the age of six continued to experience the same nightmare of persecution several times a night, during both REM and NREM sleep, nearly forty years after the event. When monitored by the EEG, long-term sufferers of nightmares are found to have shorter REM sleeps and longer REM latency than other people. Interestingly, the ability to recall our nightmares diminishes with the passage of time; perhaps such amnesia is the brain's way of trying to minimize the damage or to compensate in some way for causing disturbed sleep.

The mechanism that causes muscle paralysis during REM periods (and prevents us from acting out our dreams) sometimes breaks down. When that happens (statistically, it occurs more often in older men) the results can be funny, frightening, sometimes even tragic. For example, a friend of mine, a man in his sixties, recounted an incident in which he dreamed he was preparing to parachute from a plane. He awakened to find himself perched on a dresser about to leap to the floor, much to the consternation of his confused and understandably frightened wife. One of the sea disaster victims I mentioned above was so agitated during a dream that, even while asleep, he rose from his bed and fled from the laboratory that was attempting to monitor his sleep pattern. Approximately 85 percent of people who experience these violent dreams injure themselves. One man jumped out a window after dreaming that his house was on fire; another fell off a ladder; and another waded into a lake following a dream in which he decided to go fishing. There are even reports of patients who drive cars at high speeds as if fleeing from an attacker. According to one study, 44 percent of violent dreamers injure their bed partners, although the dreamers are not aggressive people while awake.

Children and Nightmares

As I have mentioned, nightmares occur most frequently in children, especially those who suffer from some other form of parasomnia such as bed-wetting or sleepwalking.

In children, fears of the dark or of monsters or shadows are understandable reactions to their increasing awareness of, and struggle for control over, their sometimes frightening and overpowering world. Each stage of development—learning to walk, increasing autonomy and separation from parents, toilet teaching—can trigger feelings of fear and insecurity, which can result in nightmares and other transient sleep disturbances. Also, as they grow, children develop a range of new emotions, feelings that they begin to realize can exercise a mysterious power over them and which they struggle to master. Because of the timing of these stages, nightmares are more prevalent between the ages of three and eight; at this period children are vulnerable as they grapple with the distinction between reality and fantasy. They are likely to misinterpret the shadows on the wall as horrible creatures lurking outside the bedroom. One of my patients remembered being terrified by the sight of an insect the size of a football crawling on his window. Night after night the thing appeared, until finally a stiff autumn wind blew it away. At that point, he recalled, he realized the "insect" was nothing more than the shadow of a curling oak leaf dangling from the branch of an otherwise bare tree that stood between his window and the streetlamp.

In addition to these obvious causes, children's nightmares may also be responses to their domestic situation. Parents unintentionally communicate marital, financial, or other emotional stress in more or less subtle ways—for example, by devoting less time and nurturing attention to the child. Understandably children, unable to articulate their feelings, react to these tensions in oblique ways—in some cases, through nightmares.

As a person ages, the causes of nightmares change. In late childhood or adolescence, nightmares are more likely to stem from some degree of psychopathology, such as extreme feelings of distrustfulness or alienation, or from personality traits including oversensitivity and hyperreactivity to stress. The psychological profiles of adults who suffer from nightmares twice a week or more tend to reveal schizoid personality traits. Conversely, left untreated, nightmares may actually lead to an increased risk of developing schizophrenia. Such a cause-and-effect relationship, however, is often difficult to pin down.

Nightmares may actually serve a positive function, at least to some degree, by helping the child discharge built-up emotional tension, such as resentment or fear of other people—family members or authority figures—who exercise control over the dreamer's life.

In some adolescents and adults, the use of or withdrawal from such substances as alcohol and barbiturates may also play a role in nightmares. Even one drink at bedtime can suppress REM sleep, resulting in REM rebound accompanied by disturbing dreams; after an alcoholic binge, such dreams may intrude during the waking state in the form of delirium tremens (the "DTs").

What To Do If Your Child Has Nightmares

If your child suffers from nightmares, the most important thing you can do is offer reassurance. This does not mean you should tell the child that it was "only a dream" or that the experience was not real. As far as children are concerned, such dreams *are* real. Their mental faculties are not developed to the point where they can make refined distinctions between fantasy and reality. Denying that the problem exists, or chiding them by saying that "big boys and girls aren't afraid," will not help and can actually make matters worse. Don't, for example, simply open the closet and say, "See? There's nothing there." Accept what your child is telling you; listen without judging. Show that you understand by saying such soothing things as "I can see how scary that dream was" or "I can tell you're really upset. It must have been frightening." Sometimes just by encouraging the child to talk about the dream or express the feelings accompanying it, you can help him or her to gain some measure of control over the situation. Reassurance comes when children know you will listen, understand, and accept what they tell you.

Some parents have found it effective to help the child take active steps to control the events in the dream. One father, for example, created a "magic wand" for his daughter to use to "zap the monsters" whenever they appeared. Other parents discuss with their children ways they might defeat the dragons lurking under the bed, helping them to rehearse, and thus manipulate, the outcome of the dream. Above all, do not treat children with nightmares as though they were psychologically disturbed. If the problem persists or is severe, you may wish to seek family counseling, the primary goal of which is to provide *you* with reassurance that nothing is seriously wrong with your child and that the problem will likely fade with the passage of time.

You can help the situation by taking some commonsense steps to improve the child's sleep hygiene. For example, minimize exposure to potentially troubling stimuli at bedtime. Don't read frightening stories or turn on disturbing television programs. Maintain a soothing bedtime ritual, one designed to smooth the transition to sleep in progressively relaxing stages. Use a nightlight; keep the door open so the child knows you are accessible.

Coping with Adult Nightmares

Some sleep experts advocate methods whereby sleepers train themselves to awaken as soon as a troubling dream begins, by recognizing certain settings, sounds, people, or emotions. They are urged to get out of bed, once awake, and sit calmly for a few minutes, perhaps stroking their arms or wrists as a form of neural relaxation. Another technique is to keep a dream journal, writing down the dreams immediately after waking. The simple act of writing can occupy one's mind long enough to minimize the damage from the dream; more important, perhaps, the record of dreams may help the sufferer gain insight into his or her dream patterns and reach a reconciliation with the emotional source of the nightmare.

In more severe cases some kind of insight-oriented therapy under professional guidance can be very helpful, especially when problems of fear, mistrust, or deep-seated anger are found to be the cause of nightmares. During the therapeutic process nightmares can be cast in a positive light by interpreting them as clues to the issues that tease and trouble the victim—the emotional stumbling blocks that prevent the attainment of peace of mind.

If time and counseling are insufficient, or if the problem is acute (as in cases involving overtly psychotic behavior), some form of drug therapy with antipsychotic medications may be indicated. A benzodiazepine such as clonazepam (Klonepin), also used in the treatment of nocturnal myoclonus, may help to restore the muscle-paralyzing mechanism in REM sleep. Special attention must be paid to depressed individuals, especially men, because they tend to avoid seeking professional help and are at higher risk of suicide.

NIGHT TERRORS

In England a man dreamed he was pursued by two Japanese soldiers. He strangled one—and awakened to find he had just killed his wife. The jury members were convinced by sleep experts that such events, known as night terrors, are possible, and they voted for acquittal. Fortunately for our peace of mind, such murderous calamities are rare; only two such incidents have been reported (in England, anyway) since 1960.

Night terrors (also called sleep terrors, night panics, or pavor nocturnus) are a form of parasomnia, but they are very different clinical entities from nightmares. As with a nightmare, the content of a night terror, as its name implies, is frightening. But there the similarity ends. Nightmares are the product of REM stage dreaming; night terrors, on the other hand, are arousals that occur only during the NREM stages, usually during the early part of the night—sometimes as early as fifteen minutes after the onset of sleep, but more often during Stages 3 and 4. Night terrors cause their victims to wake up screaming with intense fear. Victims' pupils are widely dilated; their hearts race at up to twice the normal rate; they sweat; they cry out for help. And although the actual night terror may last only a minute or two, its physiological effect may persist for thirty minutes or more. Because the muscle paralysis mechanism is not operating during NREM sleep, night terror victims may sit up in bed or move about the house as though fleeing from an attacker. Some people have been known to carry out complex acts, such as slashing a picture, punching through a door, or, as we have seen, assaulting a spouse. In one reported case a man pulled off the road to sleep. He experienced a night terror, which prompted him to start the car and drive away in an uncontrollable panic, eventually causing an accident that killed three people.

When the victim is able to describe a night terror attack, it is most often depicted as a single, overpowering, intensely terrifying image rather than as a narrative string of events. Usually, however, arousal following a night terror is only partial. As we have seen, victims of nightmare are usually able to recall their dreams; those who experience night terrors seldom remember having them. In the morning they may feel well rested and happy, completely unaware that, just a few hours before, they were sitting up in bed screaming in horror.

Night terrors occur primarily in children between the ages of two and five, perhaps because their central nervous systems are not yet fully developed. Fortunately, only two or three children out of a hundred (mostly boys) will experience night terrors. Children who exhibit another form of parasomnia, particularly sleepwalking, commonly suffer night terrors as well, since these disorders share many of the same pathophysiological features.

Some effects of night terror may appear to resemble an epileptic seizure—rhythmical movements of the tongue or mouth, for example. But while a form of electrical discharge or neurological disorder may underlie night terrors, they are not usually a sign that epilepsy is present. Nor are night terrors necessarily related to the presence of some form of mental disturbance or to the existence of a creative or sensitive personality, as is often the case with nightmares.

Causes of Night Terrors

What, then, causes night terrors? There may be many factors, heredity being a primary one: 96 percent of people who report night terrors have a family history of the condition. The fact that the problem begins in early childhood and usually fades by late adolescence seems to suggest that aberrations in the process of neurological maturing are involved. In some cases the presence of illness or injury—fever, brain tumor, head injury, trauma, or fatigue—may trigger an attack. Psychological factors do not usually appear to be involved in children; three out of four adults, however, report significant changes in life or levels of stress (divorce, death in the family, accident) at about the time of the attack. Also, patients sometimes report a considerable amount of pent-up anger or rage. Some psychologists attribute night terrors to a breakdown in the ego's ability to control what would otherwise be normal anxiety.

In assessing a patient who reports night terrors, I take a careful look at a number of factors: the age at which the problem began, any related stressful events, frequency and duration of the attacks, family history, and the general pattern of daytime behavior. If the family history is negative, and the terrors began after puberty, are frequent, and have persisted for a number of years, I am of course more inclined to suspect an underlying psychiatric disorder is at work, particularly if the patient seems to be maladjusted in some way. I also check for a history of fever and other sleep disorders, specifically parasomnias. In analyzing the patient's psychological profile, I quickly rule out such mental disturbances as amnesia or multiple personalities. Since night terrors are different from seizures, I watch for other signs of epilepsy. If the patient is middle-aged or elderly, I also try to rule out some underlying organic disorder, such as a brain tumor.

Possible Therapy for Night Terrors

If some psychological or organic cause of night terrors can be detected, then treatment will focus on remedying the situation. Otherwise, especially for families with children, education, reassurance, and support are usually all the treatment that is necessary. As with sleepwalking, one important practical step that can be taken is to prevent injury to the afflicted person by locking doors and windows. In adults psychiatric evaluation and appropriate treatment are called for. Rarely, I will prescribe mild benzodiazepines, such as diazepam or flurazepam, because these suppress sleep in Stages 3 and 4 and thus may have some effect for a limited time. However, drug therapy is seldom ideal for night terrors. Side effects include toxicity, habituation, drug hangover, and the possibility of interaction with alcohol, and there is a high rate of relapse of night terrors when drugs are withdrawn. The results of antidepressants such as imipramine are less certain. Such drugs, of course, are virtually never appropriate for the management of night terrors in children.

SUMMARY

While theories abound as to the reasons for and the significance of dreaming, the verdict on dreams—whether they hold the key to our inner being, or whether they will prove to be mere electrical storms, like a sort of cerebral aurora borealis—lies in the future.

Our main concern here, however, is with their effect on sleep. As we have seen, dreams on the whole are a positive, if not actually beneficial, feature of sleep. Strictly speaking, the only dream-related sleep disorders recognized by the medical profession are the ones just discussed: nightmares and night terrors. Some people who have nightmares on a regular basis may develop fears and thus experience difficulty falling asleep. Others who have conditioned themselves to awaken at the first sign of a troubling dream may be said to have a problem in maintaining sleep.

By and large, however, these are conditioned responses that can be managed relatively easily in a healthy and positive way, either through self-awareness or through psychiatric counseling, as was discussed in Chapter 10.

There is another approach that some people believe may one day prove to have merit, and that bears a brief mention here: dream control.

CAN DREAMING BE CONTROLLED?

Some people have tried—and usually failed—to influence the content of their dreams by focusing on a subject or an image just before falling asleep. However, such scenes rarely occur intact, if at all; the dreams usually undergo some sort of fragmentation or transformation.

During the last few years a number of sleep researchers have promoted various techniques known as "dream intervention" or "lucid dreaming." The concept involves supposedly training sleepers to recognize signs of dreaming: eerie landscapes or unreal patterns of color or movement, for example. By recognizing such signs and thus becoming aware they are dreaming, the sleepers can then take part in, or change the direction of, their dreams. A few people, perhaps as many as 10 percent, seem naturally able to experience lucid dreams regularly; perhaps all of us at one time or another have felt that we consciously changed the outcome of a dream.

In the laboratory, some scientists report being able to induce lucidity through use of electrical stimulation. They state that subjects can be trained to signal observers that they are having lucid dreams through such prearranged clues as eye movements, specific breathing patterns, or finger twitches. Unsurprisingly, such reports are highly controversial and have not yet been investigated in rigorous scientific fashion.

Notwithstanding, proponents of lucid dreaming claim a number of benefits deriving from the technique. For one thing, the ability to manipulate a dream consciously would reveal a great deal about the process of dreaming (and about conscious awareness itself, for that matter). Dream control could lead to a new variety of creative expression in the arts. At the very least, being able to control our dreams would enhance their value as late-night entertainment.

To medical professionals, the value of lucid dreaming would lie in its potential use as a therapeutic tool. One psychologist, for example, reported that during a dream he was being attacked by an ogre. Suddenly aware that he could control the situation, he realized the ogre was a part of himself and told the ogre that he loved it. A nightmare was thus transformed into a dream of victory over a dark and sinister force. It is perhaps possible that lucid dreaming could promote emotional healing in a limited number of patients by helping them resolve conflicts with loved ones who have died, for example, or by helping to confront—and overpower—their phobias or the demons of their past.

I must admit I am rather skeptical that lucid dreaming will prove to have much value. I am not convinced, for example, that it is wise or even safe to tamper consciously with an unconscious process, especially one so little understood as dreaming. We may cause untold damage by interfering with the basic mechanisms of dreaming, much as an untutored layman may destroy a television set by trying to fix it. (As one patient said, when told about biofeedback: "I don't want the responsibility of controlling my liver function, thank you very much.") I will reserve final judgment, however, until further controlled research into lucid dreaming is complete.

A FINAL WORD

I hope that this book has clarified for you the nature of insomnia in all its varieties and has helped to inform you of the many effective therapies that are available. The very fact that you recognize a problem exists, and have taken the step of educating yourself about it by reading books such as this, is literally half the battle. As you have seen, there is much you can do to improve your sleep habits, hygiene, and habitat. The single most important thing to remember is: THERE IS HOPE! Nothing is to be gained from continuing to suffer in silence from sleep disorders. If the commonsense strategies outlined in this book do not provide relief, then your general practitioner, family physician, or internist can recommend any number of effective pharmacological and nonpharmacological strategies that may work for you. Even if these methods fail, there are thousands of qualified sleep disorders experts, located in hundreds of hospitals and sleep research centers throughout the country, who can help. And every day new discoveries about the functions and mechanisms of sleep bring us closer to a more complete understanding of this fascinating, infuriating, mysterious, miraculous process.

Rest assured: your insomnia can be confronted—and conquered!

Appendix:
Drugs Used in the
Treatment of
Sleep Disorders

The following section contains descriptions of some of the most commonly used drugs for treating insomnia and other sleep disorders, as well as the anxiety that may accompany these sleep disorders. The drugs in this section are listed alphabetically by their chemical or generic name. If you do not know your drug's chemical name, please consult the Index.

Please note that these descriptions are provided merely as a source of information and are not intended to replace personal medical care and supervision; there is no substitute for the experience and information that a doctor can provide. In addition, the following drug profiles are in no way intended as an endorsement of these medications, nor do these profiles attempt to describe all of the drugs used in sleep disorders. If you have any questions about any medicine—either profiled or not profiled in this Appendix—please consult your doctor or pharmacist.

THE BENZODIAZEPINES

Benzodiazepines are primarily used to treat anxiety, but they may also be prescribed to treat insomnia. Among the benzodiazepines, there is little difference in overall effectiveness. The main differences among these drugs concern the length of time they remain active in the body. The shorter-acting benzodiazepines (such as lorazepam) may be good choices for people who must remain very alert during the day. Longer-acting benzodiazepines (such as diazepam) may be better for patients who need a rapid onset of action. The longer-acting drugs, however, may cause more side effects, especially daytime drowsiness. The following section contains descriptions of: diazepam, flurazepam, lorazepam, temazepam and triazolam. Other benzodiazepines not profiled include: alprazolam, chlordiazepoxide hydrochloride, clonazepam, clorazepate, dipotassium, oxazepam, halazepam, prazepam and quazepam.

**CHEMICAL NAME

Diazepam

Brand Name

Valium
T Quil
Also available in generic form.

Be Aware That:

*Long-term use of diazepam at unusually high dosages, or even at recommended-dosage levels, can cause physical addiction. Anyone who has a history of drug addiction or alcoholism may be at a greater risk of becoming physically addicted to diazepam.

*Taking diazepam with alcohol or other sedatives can cause extreme, even fatal, side effects. Because diazepam by itself may cause drowsiness, you should be careful when driving, operating machinery, or doing tasks that require concentration.

*You should not suddenly stop taking diazepam, since withdrawal symptoms such as convulsions, vomiting, muscle cramps, and sweating may result. Withdrawal from this drug should occur only under your doctor's supervision.

Tell The Doctor If:

*You have any reason to suspect you are allergic to diazepam.
*You have a history of drug or alcohol addiction.
*You are taking any prescription or over-the-counter drugs.
*You have kidney or liver disease.
*You have acute narrow-angle glaucoma.
*You are pregnant (or think you possibly might be). Because diazepam may affect your unborn baby, your doctor should not prescribe this drug unless the benefits clearly surpass any potential danger to your baby. Diazepam is not recommended for nursing mothers.

Watch Out For:

Drowsiness, fatigue, and loss of coordination. Make sure you notify your physician if any of these side effects occur. In addition, there have been reports of vivid dreams associated with the benzodiazepine class of drugs.

Drug May Interact With:

*Alcohol, monoamine oxidase (MAO) inhibitors, narcotics, barbiturates and other antidepressants, causing potentially dangerous side effects.

The Drug's Usual Dosage:

All dosages of diazepam to be established by your doctor.

**CHEMICAL NAME

Flurazepam

Brand Name

Dalmane
Also available in generic form.

Be Aware That:

*Pregnant women should not take this drug, because of potential harm to the unborn baby. Flurazepam is not recommended for nursing mothers.

*Long-term use of flurazepam at unusually high dosages, or even at recommended-dosage levels, can cause physical addiction. Anyone who has a history of drug addiction or alcoholism may be at a greater risk of becoming physically addicted to flurazepam.

*Taking flurazepam with alcohol or other sedatives can cause extreme, even fatal, side effects. Because flurazepam by itself may cause drowsiness, you should be careful when driving, operating machinery, or doing tasks that require concentration.

*This drug may cause drowsiness and may interact with alcohol even the day after you take your last dose.

*You should not suddenly stop taking flurazepam, since this may cause withdrawal symptoms such as convulsions, vomiting, muscle cramps, and sweating. Withdrawal from this drug should occur only under your doctor's supervision.

Tell The Doctor If:

*You are pregnant (or think you possibly might be).

*You have any reason to suspect you are allergic to flurazepam.

*You have a history of drug or alcohol addiction.

*You are taking any prescription or over-the-counter drugs.

*You have kidney or liver disease.

*You have acute narrow-angle glaucoma.

Watch Out For:

Drowsiness, fatigue, and loss of coordination. Make sure you notify your physician if any of these side effects occurs. In addition, there have been reports of vivid dreams associated with the benzodiazepine class of drugs.

The Drug May Interact With:

*Alcohol, monoamine oxidase (MAO) inhibitors, narcotics, barbiturates and other antidepressants, causing potentially dangerous side effects.

The Drug's Usual Dosage:

Initially, for insomnia in ADULTS: 15 to 30 mg at bedtime. For insomnia in ELDERLY patients: 15 mg at bedtime. All dosages to be established by your doctor.

**CHEMICAL NAME

Lorazepam

Brand Name

Ativan
Also available in generic form.

Be Aware That:

*Long-term use of lorazepam at unusually high dosages, or even at recommended-dosage levels, can cause physical addiction. Anyone who has a history of drug addiction or alcoholism may be at a greater risk of becoming physically addicted to lorazepam.

*Taking lorazepam with alcohol or other sedatives can cause extreme, even fatal, side effects. Because lorazepam by itself may cause drowsiness, you should be careful when driving, operating machinery, or doing tasks that require concentration.

*You should not suddenly stop taking lorazepam, since this may cause withdrawal symptoms, such as convulsions, vomiting, muscle cramps, and sweating. Withdrawal from this drug should occur only under your doctor's supervision.

Tell The Doctor If:

*You have any reason to suspect you are allergic to lorazepam.
*You have a history of drug or alcohol addiction.
*You are pregnant (or think you possibly might be). Because lorazepam may affect your unborn baby, your doctor should not prescribe this drug unless the benefits clearly surpass any potential danger to your baby. Lorazepam is not recommended for nursing mothers.
*You are taking any prescription or over-the-counter drugs.
*You have kidney or liver disease.
*You have acute narrow-angle glaucoma.

Watch Out For:

Drowsiness, fatigue, and loss of coordination. Make sure you notify your physician if any of these side effects occurs. In addition, there have been reports of vivid dreams associated with the benzodiazepine class of drugs.

The Drug May Interact With:

*Alcohol, narcotics, other antidepressants, barbiturates, MAO inhibitors and antihistamines, causing potentially dangerous side effects.

The Drug's Usual Dosage:

Initially, for insomnia in ADULTS: a single dose of 2 to 4 mg, given at bedtime. Initially, for the ELDERLY patient: One-half the usual adult dosage. All dosages to be established by your doctor.

**CHEMICAL NAME

Temazepam

Brand Name

Restoril

Be Aware That:

*Pregnant women should not take temazepam, because of potential harm to the unborn baby. Temazepam is not recommended for nursing mothers.

*Long-term use of temazepam at unusually high dosages, or even at recommended-dosage levels, can cause physical addiction. Anyone who has a history of drug addiction or alcoholism may be at a greater risk of becoming physically addicted to temazepam.

*Taking temazepam with alcohol or other sedatives can cause extreme, even fatal, side effects. Because temazepam by itself causes drowsiness, you should be careful when driving, operating machinery, or doing any task that requires concentration.

*You should not suddenly stop taking temazepam, since this may cause withdrawal symptoms, such as convulsions, vomiting, muscle cramps, and sweating. Withdrawal from this drug should occur only under your doctor's supervision.

Tell The Doctor If:

*You are pregnant (or think you possibly might be).
*You have any reason to suspect you are allergic to temazepam.
*You have a history of drug or alcohol addiction.
*You are taking any prescription or over-the-counter drugs.
*You have kidney or liver disease.
*You have acute narrow-angle glaucoma.

Watch Out For:

Drowsiness, fatigue, and loss of coordination. Make sure you notify your physician if any of these side effects occurs. In addition, there have been reports of vivid dreams associated with the benzodiazepine class of drugs.

The Drug May Interact With:

*Alcohol, monoamine oxidase (MAO) inhibitors, narcotics, barbiturates and other antidepressants, causing potentially dangerous side effects.

The Drug's Usual Dosage:

Initially, for insomnia in ADULTS: 15 to 30 mg at bedtime.
Initially, for insomnia in the ELDERLY: 15 mg at bedtime. All
dosages to be established by your doctor.

**CHEMICAL NAME

Triazolam

Brand Name

Halcion

Be Aware That:

*Long-term use of triazolam at unusually high dosages, or
even at recommended-dosage levels, can cause physical addiction. Anyone who has a history of drug addiction or alcoholism
may be at a greater risk of becoming physically addicted to
triazolam.

*Taking triazolam with alcohol or other sedatives can cause
extreme, even fatal, side effects. Because triazolam by itself may
cause drowsiness, you should be careful when driving, operating
machinery, or doing tasks that require concentration.

*You should not suddenly stop taking triazolam, since this
may cause withdrawal symptoms, such as convulsions, vomiting,
muscle cramps, and sweating. Withdrawal from this drug should
occur only under your doctor's supervision.

Tell The Doctor If:

*You have any reason to suspect you are allergic to triazolam.
*You have a history of drug or alcohol addiction.
*You are taking any prescription or over-the-counter drugs.
*You have kidney or liver disease.
*You have acute narrow-angle glaucoma.
*You are pregnant (or think you possibly might be). Pregnant

women should not use triazolam, because of the potential risks to the unborn baby. Triazolam is not recommended for nursing mothers.

Watch Out For:

Drowsiness, fatigue, memory loss, and loss of coordination. Make sure you notify your physician if any of these side effects occurs. In addition, there have been reports of vivid dreams associated with the benzodiazepine class of drugs.

The Drug May Interact With:

*Alcohol, monoamine oxidase (MAO) inhibitors, narcotics, barbiturates and other antidepressants, causing potentially dangerous side effects.

The Drug's Usual Dosage:

Initially, for ADULTS: 0.25 to 0.5 mg before bedtime. For the ELDERLY, initially: 0.125 mg at bedtime; later this dosage may be increased if necessary to 0.25 mg. All dosages to be established by your doctor.

OTHER SLEEP-INDUCING MEDICATIONS

Ethchlorvynol
Glutethimide
Both ethchlorvynol and glutethimide are classified as oral hypnotics (or sleep-inducing medications), used in the short-term treatment of insomnia.

While some physicians may use ethchlorvynol and glutethimide to treat anxiety, these drugs should be considered only after other medications (such as the benzodiazepines) have been tried.

**CHEMICAL NAME

Ethchlorvynol

Brand Name

Placidyl

Be Aware That:

*Long-term, uninterrupted use of ethchlorvynol, even at rec-
ommended-dosage levels, can cause addiction. Anyone who has
a history of drug addiction or alcoholism may be at a greater risk
of becoming addicted to ethchlorvynol.

*Taking ethchlorvynol with alcohol or other sedatives can
cause extreme, even fatal, side effects. Because ethchlorvynol
by itself may cause drowsiness, you should be careful when
driving, operating machinery, or doing tasks that require concentration.

*You should not suddenly stop taking ethchlorvynol, because
serious side effects (such as convulsions) may occur. Stop taking
this drug ONLY under your doctor's supervision.

*Pregnant women should use ethchlorvynol only when the
benefits of drug therapy clearly surpass any potential hazards
to the unborn baby. Nursing mothers should use ethchlorvynol
only with caution and only under the supervision of a physician.

*Children may become agitated or excited when taking eth-
chlorvynol.

Tell The Doctor If:

*You have any reason to suspect you are allergic to ethchlor-
vynol.

*You are pregnant (or think you possibly might be).

*You have a history of drug or alcohol addiction.

*You are taking any prescription or over-the-counter drugs.

*You have a history of porphyria (a rare blood disorder) or
kidney or liver disease.

Watch Out For:

High blood pressure, agitation, dizziness, blurred vision, morning hangover, nausea, vomiting, aftertaste, facial numbness, skin rash or shaky, uncoordinated movement. Make sure you notify your physician if any of these side effects occurs.

The Drug May Interact With:

*Alcohol, narcotics, barbiturates, and MAO inhibitors, intensifying their effects, and causing potentially dangerous, even fatal, reactions.

*Anticoagulants, decreasing their effectiveness.

*Tricyclic antidepressants, such as amitriptyline, possibly causing delirium.

The Drug's Usual Dosage:

Initially, to induce sleep in ADULTS: from 500 mg to 1 g, taken in one dose at bedtime. All dosages to be established by your doctor.

**CHEMICAL NAME

Glutethimide

Brand Name

Doriden
Also available in generic form.

Be Aware That:

*Long-term, uninterrupted use of glutethimide even at recommended dosage levels can cause addiction. Anyone who has a history of drug addiction or alcoholism may be at a greater risk of becoming addicted to glutethimide.

*Taking glutethimide with alcohol or other sedatives can cause extreme, even fatal, side effects. Because glutethimide by itself may cause drowsiness, you should be careful when driving, operating machinery, or doing tasks that require concentration.

*You should not suddenly stop taking this drug, because serious side effects such as convulsions may occur. Stop taking glutethimide ONLY under your doctor's supervision.

*Pregnant women should use glutethimide only when the benefits of drug therapy clearly surpass any potential hazards to the unborn baby. Nursing mothers should use glutethimide only with caution and only under the supervision of a physician.

*Children may become agitated or excited when taking glutethimide.

Tell The Doctor If:

*You are pregnant (or think you possibly might be).
*You have any reason to suspect you are allergic to glutethimide.
*You have a history of drug or alcohol addiction.
*You are taking any prescription or over-the-counter drugs.
*You have a history of porphyria (a rare blood disorder) or kidney or liver disease.

Watch Out For:

Skin rash, nausea, morning hangover, fatigue, agitation, difficulty breathing, and blurred vision. Make sure you notify your physician if any of these side effects troubles you.

The Drug May Interact With:

*Alcohol, narcotics, barbiturates, other sedatives, and antihistamines, intensifying their effects, and causing potentially dangerous, even fatal reactions.
*Anticoagulants such as Warfarin, thereby decreasing their effectiveness.

Your Drug's Usual Dosage:

Initially, to induce sleep in ADULTS: from 250 to 500 mg, taken in one dose at bedtime. All dosages to be established by your doctor.

THE TRICYCLIC ANTIDEPRESSANTS

Primarily used in the treatment of depression, tricyclic antidepressants can be used to provide relief for patients suffering from both insomnia and depression, since some of the tricyclic antidepressants may have sedative effects. However, I would not normally recommend these drugs in the treatment of insomnia without depression, unless other medications have failed. The tricyclic antidepressants profiled below are: amitriptyline, imipramine, and doxepin. Other tricyclic antidepressants not profiled include: desipramine, nortriptyline, protriptyline, trimipramine.

**CHEMICAL NAME

Amitriptyline

Brand Name

Elavil
Endep
Also available in generic form.

Be Aware That:

*Taking amitriptyline with alcohol or other sedatives can cause extreme drowsiness. Because amitriptyline by itself may cause drowsiness, you should be careful when driving, operating machinery, or doing tasks that require concentration.
*You should not suddenly stop taking amitriptyline.
*People over 60 may become confused when they begin taking this drug. The elderly should have regular heart examinations while taking amitriptyline.

Tell The Doctor If:

*You have any reason to suspect you are allergic to amitriptyline.

*You are recovering from a recent heart attack.
*You have a history of convulsive disorders, such as epilepsy.
*You have trouble urinating.
*You have narrow-angle glaucoma.
*You have thyroid, liver or heart disease.
*You are taking any over-the-counter or prescription drugs.
*You are pregnant (or think you possibly might be). Since amitriptyline could affect your unborn baby, your doctor should not prescribe this drug unless the benefits clearly surpass any potential dangers to the unborn baby. Amitriptyline is not recommended for nursing mothers.

Watch Out For:

Drowsiness, blurred vision, dry mouth, constipation, dizziness, rapid pulse, and difficulty urinating. Make sure you notify your physician if any of these side effects occurs.

The Drug May Interact With:

*Monoamine oxidase (MAO) inhibitors, possibly causing high fevers, high blood pressure, convulsions, and death. Don't take amitriptyline until at least two weeks after you have stopped taking MAO inhibitors.
*Alcohol and other sedatives, possibly causing extreme drowsiness.
*Ethchlorvynol (Placidyl) and disulfiram (Antabuse), possibly causing delirium.
*Antipsychotics and anticonvulsants, possibly causing the need to readjust your amitriptyline dosage.
Only with extreme caution should amitriptyline be used together with amphetamines, antihypertensive drugs, and thyroid medications.

The Drug's Dosage:

Amitriptyline is not recommended for children under 12 years old. All dosages to be established by your doctor.

**CHEMICAL NAME

Doxepin

Brand Name

Adapin
Sinequan
Also available in generic form.

Be Aware That:

*Taking doxepin with alcohol or other sedatives can cause extreme drowsiness. Because doxepin by itself may cause drowsiness, you should be careful when driving, operating machinery, or doing tasks that require concentration.

*You should not suddenly stop taking doxepin.

*People over 60 may become confused when they begin taking this drug. The elderly should have regular heart examinations while taking doxepin.

Tell The Doctor If:

*You have any reason to suspect you are allergic to doxepin.
*You are recovering from a recent heart attack.
*You have a history of convulsive disorders, such as epilepsy.
*You have trouble urinating.
*You have narrow-angle glaucoma.
*You are taking any over-the-counter or prescription drugs.
*You have thyroid, liver or heart disease.
*You are pregnant (or think you possibly might be). Since doxepin could affect your unborn baby, your doctor should not prescribe this drug unless the benefits clearly outweigh any potential dangers to your baby. Doxepin is not recommended for nursing mothers.

Watch Out For:

Drowsiness, dizziness, blurred vision, dry mouth, constipation, increased heart rate, and difficulty urinating. Make sure you notify your physician if any of these side effects occurs.

The Drug May Interact With:

*Monoamine oxidase (MAO) inhibitors, possibly causing high fevers, high blood pressure, convulsions, and death. Don't take doxepin until at least two weeks after you have stopped taking MAO inhibitors.

*Alcohol and other sedatives, possibly causing extreme drowsiness.

*Placidyl, possibly causing delirium.

*Amphetamines, antihypertensive drugs, and thyroid medications; only with extreme caution should doxepin be used together with these drugs.

The Drug's Usual Dosage:

Doxepin is not recommended for children under 12 years old. All dosages to be established by your doctor.

**CHEMICAL NAME

Imipramine hydrochloride

Brand Name

Janimine
Tofranil
Also available in generic form.

Be Aware That:

*Taking imipramine hydrochloride with alcohol or other sedatives can cause extreme drowsiness. Because imipramine hydrochloride by itself may cause drowsiness, you should be careful when driving, operating machinery, or doing tasks that require concentration.

*You should not suddenly stop taking imipramine hydrochloride.

*People over 60 may become confused when they begin taking this drug. The elderly should have regular heart examinations while taking imipramine hydrochloride.

Tell The Doctor If:

*You have any reason to suspect you are allergic to imipramine hydrochloride.

*You are recovering from a recent heart attack.

*You have a history of convulsive disorders, such as epilepsy.

*You have trouble urinating.

*You have narrow-angle glaucoma.

*You are taking any over-the-counter or prescription drugs.

*You have thyroid, liver or heart disease.

*You are pregnant (or think you possibly might be). Since imipramine hydrochloride could affect your unborn baby, your doctor should not prescribe this drug unless the benefits clearly outweigh any potential dangers to your baby. Imipramine hydrochloride is not recommended for nursing mothers.

Watch Out For:

Drowsiness, blurred vision, dry mouth, constipation, dizziness, increased heart rate, and difficulty urinating. Make sure you notify your physician if any of these side effects occurs.

The Drug May Interact With:

*Monoamine oxidase (MAO) inhibitors, possibly causing high fevers, high blood pressure, convulsions, and death. Don't take imipramine hydrochloride until at least two weeks after you have stopped taking MAO inhibitors.

*Alcohol, possibly causing extreme drowsiness.

*Ethchlorvynol (Placidyl), possibly causing delirium.

*Amphetamines, antihypertensive drugs, and thyroid medications; ONLY with extreme caution can imipramine hydrochloride be used together with these drugs.

The Drug's Usual Dosage:

For bed-wetting in CHILDREN aged 6 or older: an initial dose of 25 mg/day, to be given one hour before bedtime. If this dosage isn't effective within one week, it may be increased to 50 mg nightly for children under 12 years old. For CHILDREN over 12 years old: up to 75 mg, to be taken nightly. Dosages for children should not exceed 2.5 mg/kg daily. For ADULTS, dosages should not exceed 200 mg daily. All dosages of imipramine hydrochloride to be established by your doctor.

Bibliography

American Medical Association. *AMA Drug Evaluation Guide,* 2nd Edition, 1986.

American Psychiatric Association. *Psychiatry Update,* vol. 4. Washington: American Psychiatric Press, 1985.

Anonymous. "Apnea-hypertension link reinforced." *Medical World News,* Aug. 12 1985:83.

Anonymous. "Drugs and insomnia: the use of medications to promote sleep." *JAMA,* May 11 1984;251(18):2410–2414.

Anonymous. "How long is the night: managing insomniacs goes far beyond drugs." *Psychiatric News,* Aug. 21 1987:22–23.

Anonymous. "Jet-lag: far-reaching consequences of rapid time zone crossings." Sleep Science Information Center, Jan. 1988.

Anonymous. "The mystery of sleep." *Newsweek,* July 13 1981:48–53.

Anonymous. "Questions and answers on jet lag: interview with pioneer sleep researcher William C. Dement, M.D., Ph.D." Sleep Science Information Center, Jan. 1988.

Anonymous. "Researchers probe REM sleep and its dreams—our most puzzling nightly rituals." Sleep Science Information Center, Mar. 1987.

Anonymous. "Rhythms of life: keeping them in synch with the biological clock." Sleep Science Information Center, Oct. 1987.

Anonymous. "Study discovers incidence, severity and symptoms of jet lag." Sleep Science Information Center, Jan. 1988.

Anonymous. "Study learns how travelers cope with jet lag." Sleep Science Information Center, Jan. 1988.

Anonymous. "Throat surgery for sleep apnea is also used for snoring." *Medical World News,* Feb. 28, 1983:38–39.

Anonymous. "Waking up physicians to insomnia diagnosis." *Medical World News,* Aug. 12 1985:79–83.

Anonymous. "Why you can't sleep." *US News and World Report,* Feb. 10 1986:64–66.

Bax, M.C.O. "Sleep disturbance in the young child." *British Medical Journal,* May 10 1980:1177–9.

Biber, Michael P. "Narcolepsy." *Medical Times,* Sept. 1985;113(9):80–84.

Boffey, Philip M. "Snoring is called potentially serious health risk." *New York Times,* May 27 1986.

Borbely, Alexander. *Secrets of Sleep.* New York: Basic Books, 1986.

Boulware, Marcus H. *Snoring: New Answers to an Old Problem.* Rockaway, NJ: American Faculty Press, 1974.

Brody, Jane E. "Dreaming: a need poorly understood." *New York Times,* Aug 24, 1983:C1.

Browman, Carl P., Michael G. Sampson, Krishnareddy S. Gujavarty, Merrill M. Mitler. "The drowsy crowd." *Psychology Today,* Aug. 1982:35–38.

Burgess, Anthony. *On Going to Bed.* New York: Abbeville Press, 1982.

Busico, M. "Confronting the things that go bump in the night." Knight Ridder News Service; *The* [Bergen Co., NJ] *Record,* Feb. 29 1988:B3–4.

Candler, Thomas Oswald. "British GP reviews insomnia treatment—past and present." *Patient Care,* Mar. 30 1981:14.

Cohn, Martin A. "Fragmented sleep—a hidden health hazard." Sleep Science Information Center, July 1987.

Crystal, Howard. "Sleep disturbances in Alzheimer's disease compound families' struggle to keep loved ones at home." Sleep Science Information Center, Mar. 1987.

Demarest, Colleen B. "Helping your patient get some sleep." *Patient Care,* Feb. 15 1986:61–71.

Demarest, Colleen B. "An office workup for sleep disorders." *Patient Care,* Jan. 30 1986:20–37.

Dement, William C. "Medical community is awakening to seriousness of sleep disorders." Sleep Science Information Center, Jan. 1987.

Dement, William C. *Some Must Watch While Some Must Sleep.* San Francisco: San Francisco Book Company, Inc., 1976.

The Diagram Group: *The Brain: A User's Manual.* New York: Berkley Publishing Co., 1983.

Epstein, A. W. "Obligatory associations: a function of dreaming." *American Journal of Psychiatry,* Mar. 1988;145(3):365–66.

Erman, Milton K. "Guidelines for recognizing and treating hypersomnias." *Drug Therapy,* Aug. 1984:64–73.

Erman, Milton K. "Insomnia: treatment approaches." *Drug Therapy,* Aug. 1984:43–58.

Erman, Milton K. "Recipe for sound sleep: alcohol not an ingredient." Sleep Science Information Center, Jan. 1986.

Evans, Frederick J. "Sleep disorders and insomnia: causes and cures." *Carrier Foundation Letter #129,* Nov. 1987.

Feinsilver, Steven H. "Recognizing and treating the sleep apnea syndromes." *Emergency Medicine,* June 15, 1987:147.

Ferber, R. "Sleep, sleeplessness, and sleep disruptions in infants and young children." *Annals of Clinical Research,* 1985;17:227–234.

Folkard, Simon. "Our diurnal nature." *British Medical Journal,* Nov. 15 1986;293:1257–8.

Fry, June M. "Sleep disorders." *Medical Clinics of North America,* Jan. 1987;71(1):95–110.

Gillin, J. Christian. "Common myths about sleep and the elderly."
Sleep Science Information Center, Aug. 1987.

Gillin, J. Christian. "Sleep hygiene: battling insomnia armed with
good habits." Sleep Science Information Center, May 1986.

Gillin, J. Christian.   "Sleeping pills: when are they a safe answer for
those who can't sleep?" Sleep Science Information Center, July 1986.

Gleeson, Kevin, and Clifford W. Zwillich.   "Therapeutic approach to
obstructive sleep apnea." *Practical Cardiology,* Oct. 17 1987;13(12):55–
63.

Goldstein,   Cynthia. "Chronic   insomnia: 'multidimensional   in
cause.' " *JAMA,* Sept. 6 1985;254(9):1126–31.

Goleman, Daniel. "Do dreams really have meaning?" *New York
Times,* July 10 1984:C1.

Goleman, Daniel.   "Nightmares are linked to creativity in new view."
New York Times, Oct. 23 1984:C1.

Gross, Paul T.   "Evaluation of sleep disorders." *Medical Clinics of
North America,* Nov. 1986;70(6):1349–1360.

Hales, Dianne.   *The Complete Book of Sleep: How Your Nights Affect
Your Days.* Reading, Mass.: Addison-Wesley Publishing Co., 1981.

Hall, Jesse B. "The cardiopulmonary failure of sleep-disordered
breathing." *JAMA,* Feb. 21, 1986;255(7):930–933.

Hartmann, Ernest.   *The Sleep Book.* Washington: AARP, 1987.

Hartmann, Ernest.   "The strangest sleep disorder." *Psychology Today,*
Apr. 1981:14–18.

Hastings, A. Waller.   "The emerging science of defining and treating
sleep disturbances." *Therapaeia,* Jan. 1982:9–23.

Hearne, K.   "Control your own dreams." *New Scientist,* Sept. 24 1981:
783–5.

Hefez, A., L. Metz, and P. Lavie.   "Long-term effects of extreme situation stress on sleep and dreaming." *American Journal of Psychiatry,*
Mar. 1987;144(3):344–347.

Hetzel, M. R.   "The pulmonary clock." *Thorax,* 1981;36:481–6.

Horne, Jim.   "Warning: snoring can damage your health." *New Scientist,* Dec. 12 1985:46–48.

Horne, Jim. "Why do we need to sleep?" *New Scientist,* Nov. 12 1981: 429–31.

Hudson, L. *Night Life: The Interpretation of Dreams.* New York: St. Martin's Press, 1985.

Jacobs, E. A., C. F. Reynolds III, D. J. Kupfer, et al. "The role of polysomnography in the differential diagnosis of chronic insomnia." *American Journal of Psychiatry,* Mar. 1988;145(3):346–49.

Kales, A., E. O. Bixler, A. Vela-Bueno, et al. "Biopsychobehavioral correlates of insomnia, III: Polygraphic findings of sleep difficulty and their relationship to psychopathology." *International Journal of Neuroscience* 1984;23:43–56.

Kales, Anthony, and Joyce D. Kales. *Evaluation and Treatment of Insomnia.* New York: Oxford University Press, 1984.

Kales, Anthony, Constantin R. Soldatos, and Joyce D. Kales. "Sleep disorders: insomnia, sleepwalking, night terrors, nightmares, and enuresis." *Annals of Internal Medicine* 1987;106:582–592.

Kupfer, David J. "The 'graying' of sleep: sleep disorders grow more prevalent with age." Sleep Science Information Center, Oct. 1986.

Lamberg, Lynne. "Causes of, therapies for insomnia, other sleep problems under study." *JAMA,* Sept. 6 1985;254(9):1125–1132.

Lamberg, Lynne. "Newly awakened interest in sleep research spans many specialties." *JAMA,* Sept. 13 1985;254(10):1275–84.

Lamberg, Lynne. "A rescue kit for insomniacs." *American Health,* Mar. 1986:58–66.

Long, M. E. "What is this thing called sleep?" *National Geographic,* Dec. 1987:787–821.

Minors, D. S. "Chronobiology: its importance in clinical medicine." *Clinical Science* 1985;69:369–376.

Mitler, Merrill M. "Asleep at the wheel: a national nightmare." Sleep Science Information Center, May 1987.

Mitler, Merrill M. "Excessive daytime sleepiness: a shroud of lethargy." Sleep Science Information Center, Apr. 1986.

Montplaisir, J., J. Walsh, and J. L. Malo. "Nocturnal asthma: features of attacks, sleep and breathing patterns." *American Review of Respiratory Diseases* 1982;125:18–22.

Moore-Ede, M. C., C. A. Czeisler, and G. S. Richardson. "Circadian timekeeping in health and disease: part 1. Basic properties of circadian pacemakers." *New England Journal of Medicine,* Aug. 25, 1983; 309(8):469–476.

Morris, J. *The Dream Workbook.* New York: Fawcett Crest, 1987.

Nahmia, Jeffrey S., and Monroe S. Karetzky. "Current concepts in sleep apnea." *New Jersey Medicine,* July 1987;84(7):475–479.

Parkes, J. D. *Sleep and Its Disorders.* London: W. D. Saunders Co., 1985.

Raymond, Chris Anne: "Popular, yes, but jury still out on apnea surgery." *JAMA,* July 25, 1986;256(4):439–440.

Reynolds, Charles F. III, and David J. Kupfer. "Sleep research in affective illness: state of the art circa 1987." *Sleep,* 1987;10(3):199–215.

Roth, Thomas. "Globe-trotting and shift work: turning night into day." Sleep Science Information Center, Mar. 1986.

Schatzman, Morton. "To sleep, perchance to kill." *New Scientist,* June 1986:60–62.

Schwartz, Alice K., and Norma S. Aaron. "In quest of sleep." *New York,* Feb. 19 1979:45–52.

Tisdale, S. "The other side of midnight." *Hippocrates,* Mar.–Apr. 1988:41–52.

Upjohn Company: "What you should know about insomnia." (Brochure.) Feb. 1986.

Wortis, Joseph. "What is sleep?" *Biological Psychiatry,* 1987;22:931–932.

Zetin, Mark, Steven Potkin, and Melanie Urbanchek. "Melatonin in depression." *Psychiatric Annals,* Oct. 19 1987;17:676–81.

Index